'This is an outstandingly interesting book by Patrick Holford on a subject which is perforce of growing importance to all of us as the expectation of life increases. We need to achieve not only extra years.

sensible physical and mental exercise coupled with attention to an optimum diet which Patrick Holford explains, we can significantly reduce the mental deterioration of age.'
Dr John Marks, Life Fellow and former Director of Medical Studies, University of Cambridge

'This is an immensely important area for the public mental health of our ageing nation and this sensible approach to the prevention of Alzheimer's is to be highly recommended. Future research into these approaches should also be a high priority.'
André Tylee, Professor of Primary Care Mental Health, Institute of Psychiatry, London

'We are on the threshold of an exciting new era in preventative medicine, and Patrick Holford's comprehensive prevention plan for Alzheimer's is a sensible step forward.'
Dr Andrew McCaddon MD, GP and Honorary Research Fellow of the University of Wales College of Medicine

'It is time we woke up to the fact that Alzheimer's is a preventable disease, not an inevitable part of ageing. Just as there is nothing inevitable about heart disease, there is nothing inevitable about Alzheimer's disease. Patrick Holford's book takes up this theme with zest and is to be greatly welcomed. Each of us needs to know that Alzheimer's disease can be prevented and governments need to recognise this too. The lesson to be learnt from this book is that we can help ourselves and our loved ones by starting to modify the way we live so that our chance of developing diseases like heart disease and Alzheimer's disease is greatly reduced. But we need to begin now: the disease process begins early in life, and already in our thirties some of us have signs of Alzheimer's disease in the brain, just as we have at
Professor

BREAKING NEWS

Since this edition of the book was first reprinted, a major review of 247 studies has examined to what extent dealing with each risk factor could reduce Alzheimer's incidence. It concluded that 'Higher homocysteine levels, lower educational attainment, and decreased physical activity were particularly strong predictors.'[1] Having a high versus a low homocysteine level accounted for 22 per cent of Alzheimer's cases, while having a low versus a high intake of fish or omega-3 fats also accounted for 22 per cent of cases. The authors estimate that 'on average, one in five to one in three cases of Alzheimer's disease can potentially be averted if those risk factors were eliminated from populations'.

The systematic review and meta-analysis study, by staff scientist May Beydoun and colleagues at the US National Institute on Aging, was validated almost immediately by a British-led review in The Lancet Neurology journal. It also concluded that 'around a third of Alzheimer's diseases cases worldwide might be attributable to potentially modifiable risk factors'.[2] Unlike the Beydoun paper, it did not also assess homocysteine levels, nor intake of fish or omega-3 status, so could make no comment on these risk factors. However, for those factors assessed by both research groups (education, physical inactivity and smoking) the conclusions are the same – Alzheimer's is largely preventable and a diet- and lifestyle-related disease. That is the message of this book.

1. Beydoun M. A., Beydoun H. A., Gamaldo A. A. et al., 'Epidemiologic studies of modifiable factors associated with cognition and dementia: systematic review and meta-analysis', *BMC Public Health*, 14(1):643 (2014).
2. Sam N. et al., 'Potential for primary prevention of Alzheimer's disease: an analysis of population-based data', *Lancet Neurol*, 13:788–94 (2014).

patrick

HOLFORD

with Shane Heaton & Deborah Colson

THE ALZHEIMER'S PREVENTION PLAN

10 PROVEN WAYS TO STOP MEMORY DECLINE AND REDUCE THE RISK OF ALZHEIMER'S

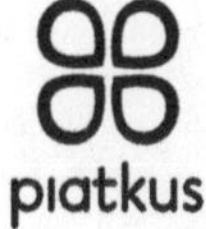

First published in Great Britain in 2005 by Piatkus Books
Reprinted 2007

This updated and expanded version first published 2011
Reprinted 2011, 2013, 2014

A CIP catalogue record for this book
is available from the British Library.

ISBN 978-0-7499-2514-7

Typeset in Minion by Phoenix Photosetting, Chatham, Kent
Printed and bound in Great Britain by CPI Group (UK) Ltd, Croydon, CR0 4YY

Papers used by Piatkus are natural, renewable and recyclable
products sourced from well-managed forests and certified
in accordance with the rules of the Forest Stewardship Council.

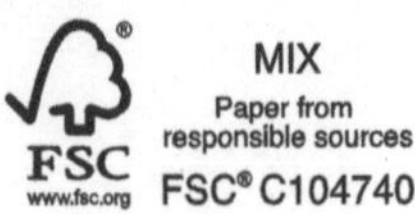

Piatkus
An imprint of
Little, Brown Book Group
100 Victoria Embankment
London EC4Y 0DY

An Hachette UK Company
www.hachette.co.uk

www.piatkus.co.uk

About the author

Patrick Holford BSc, DipION, FBANT, CNHCRP is a leading spokesman on nutrition in the media, specialising in the field of mental health. He is author of over 30 books, translated into more than 20 languages and selling over a million copies worldwide, including the *Optimum Nutrition Bible* and *Optimum Nutrition for the Mind.*

Patrick Holford started his academic career in the field of psychology. In 1984 he founded the Institute for Optimum Nutrition (ION), an independent educational charity, and was involved in groundbreaking research showing that multivitamins can increase children's IQ scores – research that was published in the *Lancet* and was the subject of a *Horizon* documentary in the 1980s. He was one of the first promoters of the importance of zinc, antioxidants, essential fats, low-GL diets and homocysteine-lowering B vitamins such as folic acid.

He is chief executive of the Food for the Brain Foundation and director of the Brain Bio Centre, the Foundation's treatment centre. He is also an honorary fellow of the British Association of Applied Nutrition and Nutritional Therapy, and a member of the Nutrition Therapy Council.

Disclaimer

Mental health is a complex affair. While all the nutrients and herbs referred to in this book have been proven safe, those seeking help are advised to consult a qualified clinical nutritionist or health professional who can run the necessary tests and is informed about drug–nutrient interactions. The recommendations given in this book are intended solely for educational and information purposes and not as medical advice. Neither the author nor the publisher accept liability for readers who choose to self-prescribe.

All supplements should be kept out of reach of infants and young children.

Foreword

Time wastes all things, the mind too: often I remember how in boyhood I outwore long sunlit days in singing; now I have forgotten so many a song.

Virgil, Eclogue IX
(translated by J. W. Mackail)

Virgil, one of the great poets of ancient Rome, may have been writing 2,000 years ago – but even then it was recognised that our memory begins to fade as we age. Today we are seeing the phenomenon in alarming numbers: every year over a million elderly people in Europe and about 750,000 in the US and Canada begin to suffer from memory loss. The latest estimates indicate that there are some 5 million elderly in the USA with memory impairment and 14 million in greater Europe. Within five years, at least half and possibly as many as 70 per cent of people with impaired memory will go on to develop dementia, the most common form of which is Alzheimer's disease.

The World Health Organization has estimated that in 2000, the total number of people with dementia stood at 22 million.

Given our ageing world population, it's likely that by 2050, some 114 million people will have Alzheimer's disease.

Dementia is a huge and growing epidemic. But what can we do about it? Are any governments planning to tackle it? And are the major drug companies developing new treatments for combating it? The answer is no – at least, not with any great sense of urgency or vision.

This startling indifference to an urgent international problem begs another question: why? I think the main reason is that a kind of fatalism has arisen over Alzheimer's disease. For centuries people have believed, like Virgil, that a decline in memory is an inevitable part of ageing and that, since memory loss is the cardinal symptom of Alzheimer's disease, it too is inevitable.

This idea has become dogma, but it is wrong. Alzheimer's disease is not an inevitable part of ageing. It is a true disease. But a second dogma has also emerged around Alzheimer's: that it can all be explained by our genes, making it impossible for certain people to escape it. Once again, this is not true. A mere fraction of people with Alzheimer's disease, perhaps only 1 per cent, develop the condition only because of mutations in certain genes.

Most cases of Alzheimer's disease are caused by a combination of many different factors coming together in the same person. Some of these so-called 'risk factors' are genetic, but these mutations are not deterministic and their effect can be influenced by a large number of non-genetic risk factors, one of which is increasing age. Now, the important thing is that many of the non-genetic risk-factors can be modified. We can, for example, change our lifestyle or our diet. In so doing, we can greatly reduce the risk of developing diseases like heart disease. Heart disease and stroke have declined almost to half in developed countries in the last 50 years, and this is in large part due to the recognition that they are multifactorial diseases, with many different non-genetic risk factors. Smoking, for example, is a major risk factor for diseases of the blood vessels, and the drop in smoking has made a major contribution to the drop in deaths from heart disease and stroke.

And just as there is nothing inevitable about heart disease, there is nothing inevitable about Alzheimer's. Patrick Holford's book takes up this theme with zest and is to be greatly welcomed. It covers recent research – including my own studies with the OPTIMA team at the University of Oxford – that is providing exciting evidence that life-style factors, including diet, may have a strong influence on the risk of dementia. Each of us needs to know that Alzheimer's disease can be prevented and governments need to recognise this too. The lesson to be learnt from this book is that we can help ourselves and our loved ones by starting to modify the way we live so that our chance of developing Alzheimer's disease is greatly reduced. But we need to begin now: the disease process begins early in life, and even in our thirties, some of us have signs of Alzheimer's disease in the brain, just as we have atherosclerosis in our blood vessels. Get started!

Professor David Smith
Professor Emeritus of Pharmacology, University of Oxford; Founding Director of Oxford Project to Investigate Memory and Ageing (OPTIMA)

Introduction

WHAT IS THE POINT of a long life if you can't remember it – and what is more tragic than losing your mind before you lose the use of your body?

This is one of those bad news/good news stories. The bad news, put simply, is that 3 in 10 people over the age of 70 have poor memory, poor concentration and confusion; 1 in 10 have dementia – a diagnosed and quite severe mental decline; and 1 in 15 have probable Alzheimer's, in which their brain is rapidly degenerating. That means that you have roughly a 50/50 chance of entering the last quarter of your life with your marbles intact.

The good news is that memory decline, dementia and even Alzheimer's are preventable. But are they 100 per cent preventable? The answer is – probably. In researching this book I have had the opportunity to speak to the top doctors and researchers in Alzheimer's and age-related cognitive decline. And without exception, that is their opinion and mine. But the time to act is NOW.

This book isn't intended only for the elderly – it was written for anyone at any age with a brain and a modicum of common sense. As you will soon realise, Alzheimer's disease is a long time coming. The first signs of brain degeneration probably begin at least 20 years before a diagnosis is made. It has all the hallmarks of other modern-day degenerative diseases, such as diabetes, cardiovascular disease and cancer. We now know that both cardiovascular disease and type 2 diabetes are largely caused by inappropriate diet, environment and lifestyle. Cancer, in general, is also at least 80 per cent due to what you do in your life, not what you inherit genetically. That was the conclusion of a study involving 44,000 twins, with identical genes but a completely different incidence of cancer.

Also, the fact that Alzheimer's incidence – much like diabetes and heart disease – varies widely from country to country, suggests it's more to do with diet and lifestyle than genes. For example, the prevalence of Alzheimer's is almost twenty times higher in Israel than India or Africa.[1]

Genes are blamed for far too much. In case you didn't know, genes don't cause disease. Genes contain the building instructions for proteins in the body. Proteins make enzymes, which do the work of turning one body chemical into another. So you can inherit a faulty enzyme system that might tip you towards diseases such as Alzheimer's. Enzymes, in turn, are activated by nutrients. In most cases, if you have a defective enzyme, you need more of specific nutrients. I'm going to show you that roughly 1 in 10 people inherit a genetic tendency towards both cardiovascular disease and Alzheimer's – and how to find out if you are one of them. If so, you will need to increase your intake of specific nutrients.

Alzheimer's and other forms of dementia are terrible diseases. Their fearsome aspect is twofold – first, in losing the sense of who you are and secondly, in not knowing what you can do about it. And based on current trends, we are going to see the number of sufferers rise to over 1 million in Britain (it is currently 820,000) and 63 million in the world over the next 25 years.[2] The burden this will place on sufferers, their families and healthcare systems will become a major problem for society. Already, dementia costs the UK alone £23 billion a year.

Yet we already know a great deal about what causes age-related memory decline and Alzheimer's. There are literally thousands of research studies that collectively point to ways of dramatically reducing your risk. What these studies show is that Alzheimer's and age-related memory decline can be prevented, but that the time to act is sooner rather than later.

If these conditions can be prevented, can they be reversed? This is a much harder question to answer at this point in time. In the case of Alzheimer's disease we are talking about damage to the brain. While the brain does rebuild, the process doesn't happen overnight. There are no studies yet that show reversal, yet there are a growing number of cases of people with probable Alzheimer's who have improved, and have not deteriorated further.

At the Brain Bio Centre in London we are applying the comprehensive approach in this book to maximise mental performance – and we are getting some extraordinary results. Prevention, however, is not only better than cure, it's a lot easier.

My hope for you and your family is that you'll read this book, put my suggestions into practice and keep your mind, memory, concentration, mood and intelligence intact throughout your life.

Wishing you the best of health.

Patrick Holford

PART 1

Why Alzheimer's and Memory Decline are Preventable

If your memory isn't as good as it used to be, your concentration is flagging and your mind is some way off sharp, you may be another victim of a widespread epidemic – brain drain. Officially called age-related memory decline, far too many people are experiencing declining cognitive function far too early. However, both memory loss and Alzheimer's disease are preventable, and in this section of the book I'll be showing you why and how.

1

How's Your Brain?

YOUR BRAIN CAN BE your greatest friend or your worst enemy. If it's working, you're able to think clearly, to imagine, to sense, to dream, to feel. It is your brain that makes you who you are. If it's not working, you can feel flat, unhappy, confused, forgetful – life loses its clarity and becomes a foggy struggle.

So how is your brain, and what are you doing to keep it healthy?

You might think this question is a little odd. But keeping your brain in shape is no stranger than servicing your car, or keeping your muscles taut or your body in trim. Why, then, do so many of us do so little to maintain the health of our brains? More than any other organ of the body, your brain is key to living a happy, fulfilling and pain-free life.

This 3–pound mass of mainly fat and water nestling in our skulls is not only the most complex and mysterious part of us. It also is the most regenerative, hardwiring a new neuronal connection every minute; and because of this, it is the most energy-expensive. On a sedentary day, your brain will consume as much as 40 per cent of all the calories you eat, and think an estimated 60,000 thoughts! More than any other organ of the body, it depends on a second-by-second supply of the right nutrients.

So, how is your brain? Is it firing on all cylinders, or is your mind less sharp and your memory less reliable than it used to be? If you'd like to pin down your cognitive state with fair precision, there are three ways to give your brain an MOT: psychological tests, physical tests and chemical tests. Let's kick off with psychological testing.

Psychological brain testing

Many people, young and old, experience memory and concentration problems. In Britain's largest ever health and diet survey, the 100% Health Survey, we asked over 55,000 people questions such as those shown below in the mind and memory check.[3] Here's what we found.

Two-thirds of the respondents suffered from anxiety, and 48 per cent reported feeling depressed. Difficulty concentrating and feeling confused was experienced by 47 per cent, 39 per cent felt nervous or hyperactive, and 39 per cent reported poor memory or difficulty learning new things.

Now check yourself out with the Mind and Memory Check questionnaire on the following page.

Mind and Memory Check

- [ ] Is your memory deteriorating?
- [ ] Do you find it hard to concentrate and often get confused?
- [ ] Do you sometimes meet someone you know quite well but can't remember their name?
- [ ] Do you often find you can remember things from the past but forget what you did yesterday?
- [ ] Do you ever forget what day of the week it is?
- [ ] Do you ever go looking for something and forget what you are looking for?
- [ ] Do your friends and family think you're getting more forgetful now than you used to be?
- [ ] Do you find it hard to add up numbers without writing them down first?
- [ ] Do you often experience mental tiredness?
- [ ] Do you find it hard to concentrate for more than an hour?
- [ ] Do you often misplace your keys?
- [ ] Do you frequently repeat yourself?
- [ ] Do you sometimes forget the point you're trying to make?
- [ ] Does it take you longer to learn things than it used to?

Score 1 for each 'yes' answer.

If your score is:

Below 5: You don't have a major problem with your memory – but you'll find that supplementing natural mind and memory boosters will sharpen you up even more.

5 to 10: Your memory definitely needs a boost – you are starting to suffer from brain drain. Follow all the diet and supplement recommendations here.

More than 10: You are experiencing significant memory decline and need to do something about it. As well as following all the diet and supplement recommendations in this chapter, see a nutritionist.

Now fill in your scores on the Your Brain's MOT chart, in Appendix 1, page 205.

Age and memory decline

If you've compared your answers to the questionnaire with the percentages in the 100% Health survey mentioned on page 7, and come out about average, you might be feeling relieved. But are you really satisfied with having an 'average' memory? My goal for you is to be better than average, and keep your mind, mood and memory razor-sharp throughout your life.

On the other hand, what if you clocked up a worrying number of 'yeses'? If you did, you're not alone. According to the drug companies, there is an epidemic of age-related memory decline. 'Age-associated memory impairment affects many more people than Alzheimer's disease, although it's certainly true that it is a much less severe condition,' says Dr Paul Williams of pharmaceuticals giant Glaxo, who have been researching drugs to enhance memory and mental performance. 'We believe at least 4 million people in the UK suffer from this.'

Age-related memory decline or 'mild cognitive impairment', as it is often called, is a long way off dementia or Alzheimer's, and there is no guarantee that one will lead to the other. However, as you will see, these milder symptoms are the first sign of potential problems later in life, and the key to prevention is to start early.

Are you concerned?

If you are worried about your own memory, or about that of a friend or relative, there are more comprehensive psychological tests that you can take. You'll find one of these, the TICS test, in Appendix 2, page 207. Without looking at this test yourself, have someone read you the questions and then score the answers. If you score below 26, you have some level of cognitive impairment and it's worth going to your doctor, as well as wholeheartedly following the Alzheimer's Prevention Diet and my recommendations for supplementation and exercise, all detailed in Part 3.

Physicals for the brain

The brain is not just a cognitive wonder, a world within a world; it's also an organ, and just like your heart or lungs, your doctor can examine it for damage. Unfortunately, this procedure is neither as easy nor as inexpensive as taking your pulse or blood pressure, so your doctor will not request a brain physical unless you are showing significant signs of memory decline.

There are three kinds of scan available, all designed to see if there are any areas of damage, abnormality or 'shrinkage'. This might sound scary, but the brain does tend to shrink with age. In fact, it's common for 20 per cent of brain cells to die over a lifetime, so that by the age of 70, most people's brains have shrunk by 10 per cent. A gradual loss of control of the complex orchestra of hormones and neurotransmitters often accompanies this shrinkage, leading to diminished brain power, slower memory retrieval, a reduced sex drive, less energy, less motivation and fewer emotional highs.

However, declining mental function is not inevitable. Surprising as it may seem, you can build new brain cells at any age, although the process is a slow one. Research clearly shows that healthy, well-educated elderly people often show no decline in mental function right up to death, and no increased rate of brain shrinkage even after the age of 65.[4]

There are three kinds of physical for the brain. Let's look at them now.

CT scan

The CT scan is the most common type of brain scan. It's a computerised 3D X-ray ('CT' stands for 'Computerised X-ray Tomography') and can pick up an area of damage, perhaps caused by a mild stroke, or a brain tumour.

MRI scan

Magnetic Resonance Imaging or MRI is a more advanced scan. When you take one of these scans you pass your head, or body, through a tube which contains a strong magnetic field. This makes the water in your cells vibrate and give off an electrical signal which is then interpreted by a computer, and turned into a map of 'slices' of your brain. Another type of scan, functional MRI, can pick up areas of the brain that use more oxygen. The more damaged an area, the less oxygen present in it.

PET and SPECT scans

Positron Emission Tomography (PET) and Single Photon Emission Computerised Tomography (SPECT) scans are currently very rarely used, and are more expensive than other types. They're reserved mainly for research, but can show similar information about the brain. They involve injecting a chemical that acts as a marker for the brain and can indicate the level of blood brain flow and the metabolic activity in different regions of the brain.

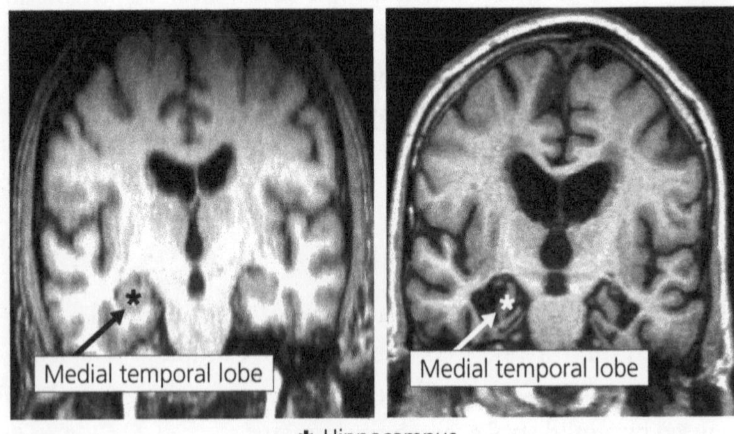

Figure 1. MRI scans of a healthy brain (left) and that of an Alzheimer's patient (right)

Basically, the healthier your brain, the better the flow of blood. As a brain cell makes energy, it needs a supply of glucose – the body's main fuel – and oxygen, plus a whole array of other brain-friendly nutrients. If a clump of your brain cells have died off, their blood supply will die off too. So, measures of both oxygen concentration (functional MRI) and blood brain flow (PET and SPECT) are the most sensitive tests currently used to find out if parts of the brain are degenerating.

What is also interesting, and just beginning to be researched, are the effects of nutrition, meditation, exercise or yoga on blood brain flow. Blood brain flow may prove to be the physical yardstick of what keeps your brain firing on all cylinders.

Needless to say, if arteries leading to the brain, such as the carotid arteries in the neck, are blocked in any way (by, for example, the 'furring up' that occurs in atherosclerosis), this will also decrease flow of blood to the brain and increase the risk of memory impairment and dementia later in life.

DIY chemical tests for the brain

While you are unlikely ever to have a brain scan, did you know you can test one of the most important indicators of brain health at home? This is your brain's chemical balance. Brain cells only die off if there's something wrong with the supply of vital chemicals, such as glucose, oxygen, vitamins, minerals and essential fats. Making sure you have an optimal supply, through diet and supplements, is a cornerstone to keeping your mind forever young.

So how do you test to see if your brain has enough of them? You'll find out how in Chapter 6, where I explain the brain foods that are essential, and need to become a part of your diet. But that is only one aspect of nourishing your brain. The flipside of the coin is to avoid the substances, which I call 'anti-nutrients', that can damage your brain. These include too much copper, mercury, lead and cadmium, but also others such as alcohol and carbon monoxide, from pollution. In Chapters 12 through to 15 I explain how to avoid them, and also introduce you to simple tests, such as hair mineral analysis, which can identify if you've got enough of the good guys, or too much of the bad guys.

There's another key test that checks to see if our brain chemistry is on an even keel, and it hinges on a critical bodily process known as methylation. The ability of the brain to make new brain cells and to make neurotransmitters – the messenger chemicals that control your mood and memory – depends on methylation. Think of it as your brain's inbuilt toolbox. There are a billion methylation events every second doing hundreds of chemical balancing acts in the brain: fixing damage, making more adrenalin, detoxifying an 'anti-nutrient'.

One chemical in the blood, an amino acid – or protein building block – known as homocysteine, determines how good you are at this methylation business. Homocysteine is to your brain like cholesterol is to your arteries. The level of it in your blood predicts, more accurately than any other chemical measure, your risk for memory, mood and concentration problems. If your level is high, you substantially increase your risk of dementia or Alzheimer's later in life.[5] That's the bad news. The good news is that it's relatively straightforward to rapidly reduce your homocysteine level and your risk, and that testing your level is easy, and involves the use of a simple home test kit. I'll tell you how to deal with homocysteine in Chapter 7 and show you the evidence that lowering it can improve your memory if you are showing signs of cognitive decline.

So there is much you can do on the chemical balance front. But to understand methylation and brain chemistry per se, you need to understand how your brain actually works.

2

How Your Brain Works

IF YOU'RE GOING TO begin looking after your brain it helps to know a little about how it actually functions. As I mentioned in Chapter 1, every day we have around 60,000 thoughts. (Most of them are repeats!) Every single thought you think triggers a 'ripple' of activity across the network of specialised nerve cells – which are known as neurons – that help to make up your brain. Here's how it works.

Each neuron links up to other neurons – and it's a prodigious network. You've got a hundred billion neurons, each connecting to thousands of others. To get an idea of just how complex that is, consider the Amazon rainforest. This ecological wonderland stretches for some 7 million square kilometres (about 2.7 million square miles) and contains about a hundred billion trees. So there are as many nerve cells in our brain as trees in the entire Amazon rainforest, and as many connections as leaves!

Neurons have 'arms' called dendrites, each of which has an axon at the end. Where one axon meets another neuron, there's a gap, like the 'spark' gap in a spark plug. This is called a synapse, and messages (which are actually chemicals known as neurotransmitters, as we'll see) are sent from one neuron to another across it.

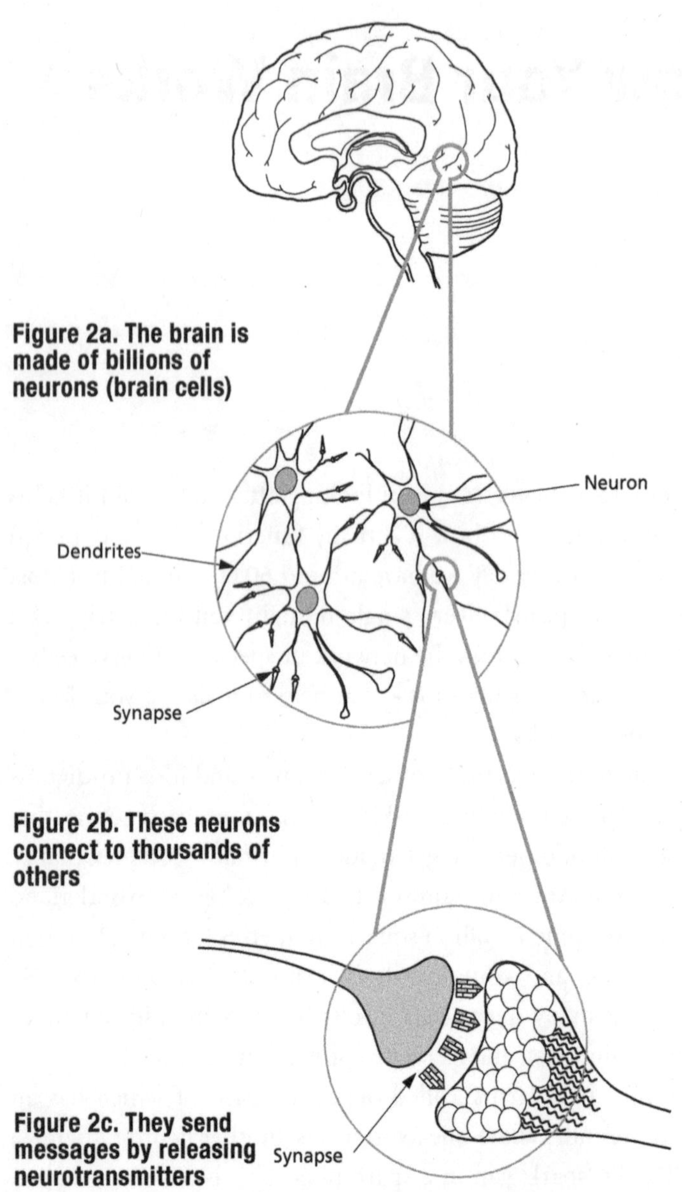

Figure 2a. The brain is made of billions of neurons (brain cells)

Figure 2b. These neurons connect to thousands of others

Figure 2c. They send messages by releasing neurotransmitters

The stations that send and receive the messages, known as receptors, are built out of essential fats which are also found in fish and seeds; phospholipids, which are abundant in eggs and organ meats; and amino acids.

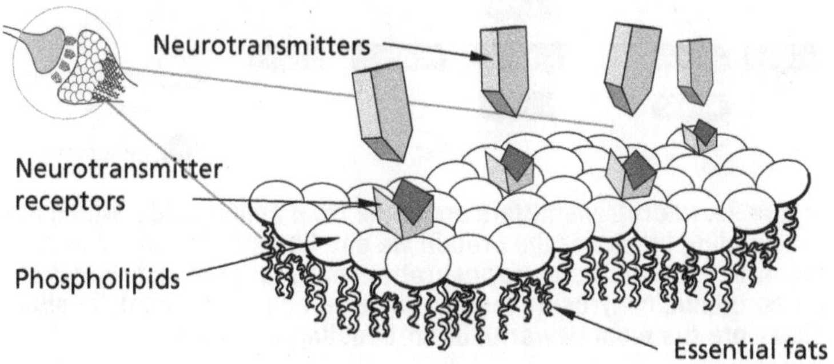

Figure 2d. These messages dock into receptor sites on neighbouring neurons

In most cases, the neurotransmitter, or 'message', is also made from amino acids or related substances. Some neurotransmitters are themselves amino acids, but different amino acids can also make different neurotransmitters. For example, the neurotransmitter serotonin, which keeps you happy, is made from the amino acid tryptophan. Adrenalin, noradrenalin and dopamine, which keep you motivated, are made from phenylalanine. And one of the key neurotransmitters responsible for memory, acetylcholine, is made from choline, found in eggs.

Turning an amino acid into a neurotransmitter is no simple job. It's done by enzymes in the brain that depend on 'intelligent' nutrients. These include vitamins, minerals and special amino acids.

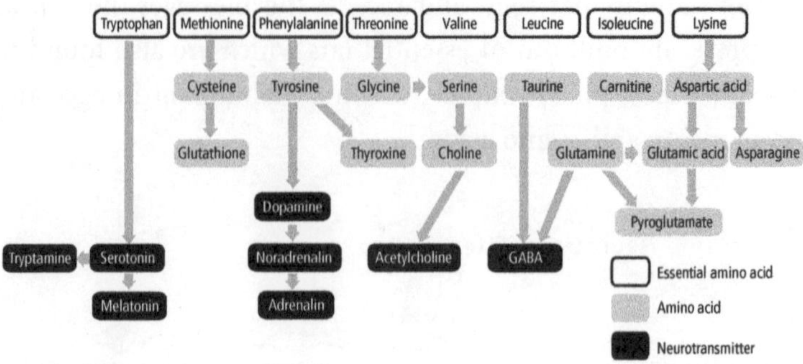

Figure 2e. Neurotransmitters are made from amino acids, which are the building blocks of the protein we eat. Specific amino acids are the direct precursors of key neurotransmitters, such as tryptophan for serotonin, or tyrosine for dopamine, or choline for acetylcholine. These are the most powerful brain-boosting nutrients

Why methylation keeps your mind sharp

We first encountered methylation in the preceding chapter. This process, and the group of nutrients involved in it, help make and keep your level of neurotransmitters well balanced, which is vital for a healthy, properly functioning brain.

To understand methylation, we need to know a bit about body chemistry. Your body is quite literally a sea of chemicals concocted out of millions of them, from glucose to fats, and amino acids to hormones and neurotransmitters.

And this chemical sea, just like the planetary ones, is constantly shifting. For example, when you are under stress, the body makes more adrenalin to keep you going. When you go to bed, the body releases melatonin to help you sleep. When you are dreaming, the body produces more acetylcholine. These are just three examples of literally hundreds of thousands of adjustments the body makes every second to keep you healthy and happy.

But how on earth does your body keep everything in balance? This is where methylation comes in. In this process, 'methyl groups'– made up of one carbon and three hydrogen atoms – are added to, or subtracted from, other molecules. This is how the body makes the substances it needs, or breaks down those it doesn't – by transforming one biochemical into another.

Methylation happens a billion times a second. It is like one big dance, with biochemicals passing methyl groups from one partner to another.

Take noradrenalin. The body produces this chemical to keep you happy and motivated. However, if you are under stress, it adds a methyl group to noradrenalin to make adrenalin, which gives you a burst of energy and aggression – the well-known 'fight or flight syndrome'.

Methyl groups come from the food you eat. For example, when you eat a piece of fish containing the amino acid methionine, it's incorporated into your bloodstream and inside your cells; then a methyl group is taken away from the methionine, leaving you with homocysteine. When everything is working well, the body adds a different methyl group back to homocysteine to convert it into an extraordinarily important chemical called S-adenosyl methionine (SAMe, pronounced 'Sammy', for short). SAMe is a natural mind and mood booster. This is because it can readily give up its methyl group to help alter other body chemicals and keep your brain in balance, or pick up other methyl groups.

If your level of homocysteine is high, this means you've got a log jam in your body and brain chemistry, and you've become a poor 'methylator'. As we shall see, this is one of the main likely causes of Alzheimer's disease. As we saw in Chapter 1, having a high level of homocysteine is not only strongly associated with an increased risk of Alzheimer's, it's also associated with declining memory and mood in general.

The well-fed brain

Throughout this chapter, I've given you hints and tips on how to feed your brain; now it's time to spell it out. Nutrients, as you'll see, are one of the greatest brain boosters, so having the right ones in your fridge and cupboard is essential for keeping mind and memory in order.

First, how can you improve that vital process, methylation, and so lower your homocysteine level? A number of nutrients will do the job: vitamins B6, B12, folic acid, as well as trimethylglycine (TMG) or SAMe (see page 19), B2, zinc and magnesium. And here's the lowdown on the rest.

For a well-fed brain, you need:

- Vitamins (especially the antioxidants A, C, D and E, and B vitamins)
- Minerals (especially zinc and magnesium)
- Essential fats (both omega-3 and 6 fatty acids)
- Phospholipids (especially phosphatidyl choline and serine)
- Amino acids (found in protein)
- Glucose (evenly supplied by less refined carbohydrate foods, such as brown rice)
- Oxygen (from the atmosphere).

And to make neurons and neurotransmitters:

- Acetylcholine
- Serotonin
- Adrenalin, noradrenalin and dopamine
- GABA.

We'll see the best ways of obtaining all these substances in Part 3. But how will you know if you're deficient in them in the first place? The chances are you're not getting nearly enough.

One way to tell is the speed of your thought processes. These nutrients not only keep your brain working well, they keep it working fast. The healthy brain of a young person processes a thought at a speed of 320 milliseconds – roughly a third of a second. People with age-related memory decline take 498 milliseconds, roughly half a second. Older people of a similar age, but with no decline in memory, will take 396 milliseconds.

So it appears that age slows thinking, but nothing like as much as the disease process that so often leads to Alzheimer's. One study, for instance, showed that those with age-related memory decline or Alzheimer's showed marked differences in mental processing speed.[6–7] And of course, it's not just the speed of your mind, but also the ability to process and store memories, that suffers in a poorly nourished brain.

In fact, not getting enough of just one nutrient can have a dramatic effect on cognitive power. In Chapter 9, for instance, you'll see how a shortfall of DHA (one of the omega-3 fats and a top brain nutrient) during pregnancy not only slows down the child's speed of thought at birth, but leaves their brain still thinking more slowly six to eight years later!

By the time you reach the end of this book, you'll know exactly what you need to do to guarantee you get an optimal supply of every single vital brain nutrient that keeps your brain thinking fast and working well.

Now that you know something about how the brain works, and the nutrients it needs, let's explore what goes wrong in Alzheimer's and dementia, so you know why it's preventable – and how to prevent it.

3

The Origin of Alzheimer's Disease

ONE OF THE MOST dangerous and incorrect assumptions often made about Alzheimer's is that it is a natural consequence of ageing – and that therefore, the longer you live, the more likely you are to develop it.

This is simply not true. Many people live to a ripe old age without any significant loss in mental faculties.[8] Only a small proportion of older people develop dementia and Alzheimer's.

In some countries, for example India and China, that proportion appears to be less than half that occurring in Britain. When people in one country suffer much more from a disease than people of a similar age in another country, this is a sure sign that the difference has something to do with diet, lifestyle or other environmental factors – or genetic variance. As you'll see, we can rule out genetic differences as the major factor, particularly because Chinese and Indian people who emigrate to Britain soon acquire a similar risk for developing dementia. So the implication is that by identifying and changing the diet and lifestyle factors that are the culprits in the case, Alzheimer's is essentially preventable.

As I've said, a decline in memory and concentration is not the same thing as a diagnosis of dementia or probable Alzheimer's, although it does mean your chances of developing these conditions are higher. Every year roughly a million people in Europe will develop age-related cognitive impairment. Within a few years, more than 50 per cent, and possibly 80 per cent, of these people will develop dementia.[9] Currently, there are an estimated 750,000 people with dementia in Britain, and some 24 million worldwide.

Roughly speaking, 50 to 70 per cent of people diagnosed with dementia will end up diagnosed with probable Alzheimer's, while 20 per cent will be given a diagnosis of vascular dementia, caused by constricted blood flow to the brain due to blocked arteries. There are other forms, such as dementia with Lewy bodies, fronto-temporal dementia (including the largely genetic Pick's disease), and dementia caused by a stroke, a bleed in the brain or a brain tumour. But as Alzheimer's is the most widespread, let's look at it in depth.

The anatomy of Alzheimer's

Dementia – including Alzheimer's – is an insidious condition. In the early stages, sufferers have increasing symptoms of absent-mindedness, low mood and an inability to learn new things. Judgement, and their ability to function intellectually and socially, begin to go awry. The person may repeatedly forget to turn off the iron, or may not recall which medicines they took in the morning. They may start to show mild personality changes, such as a lack of spontaneity or a sense of apathy and a tendency to withdraw from social interactions.

Later on, there will be a loss of logic and memory, disorientation and poor coordination. Speech deteriorates and paranoia may appear. At this point, a diagnosis of probable Alzheimer's disease may be given. Why 'probable'? Because Alzheimer's is properly diagnosed, not simply by symptoms, but by the presence of a specific kind of degeneration in a specific part of the brain – and this is difficult to see without the aid of expensive scans.

The German neuropathologist Alois Alzheimer discovered this characteristic degeneration in the brain back in 1906. Using a technique known as silver stain, he examined the brain cells of a woman who died prematurely at 55 with signs of dementia, and found a tangled mess of proteins and clusters of degenerating nerve endings, called neurofibrillary tangles. This condition is associated with a gradual dying-off of neurons and poor communication between neurons. There is also often a build-up of something called beta-amyloid plaque, a protein-like substance that shouldn't be there.

Since that time, research into Alzheimer's has continued apace. Largely thanks to the pioneering work of Professor David Smith and colleagues in the University of Oxford's pharmacology department, we now know that Alzheimer's is a specific disease process, not just a random, gradual decline in brain cells, and that it originates in a particular brain region. Their Optima (Oxford Project to Investigate Memory and Ageing) study has been running since 1988 and has proved, among other things, that the damage leading to Alzheimer's begins in a central part of the brain known as the medial temporal lobe.[10–13]

Pinpointing the problem area

The medial temporal lobe, which contains the structures known as the hippocampus and the parahippocampal gyrus, is vital for both mood and memory. Even though this lobe accounts for only 2 per cent of the brain's total area, it is essential for the processing of everything we sense, feel or think.

Precisely because it's in the middle of the head, it's a difficult

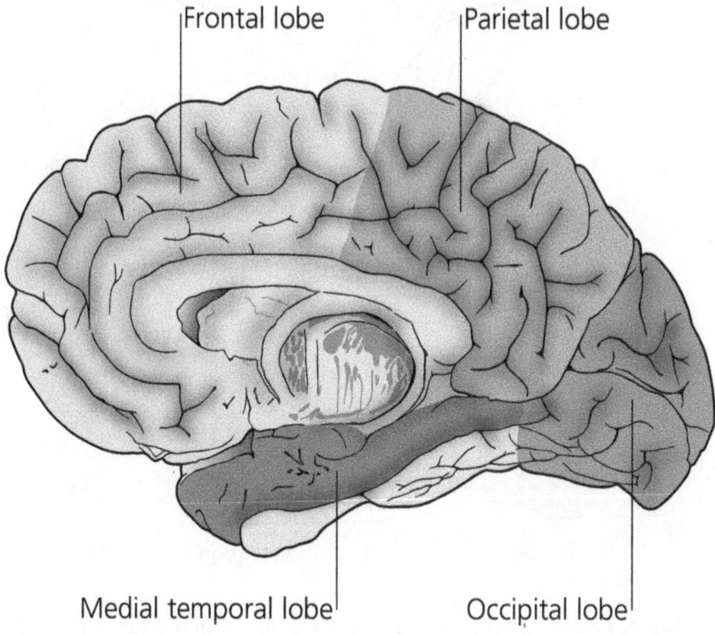

Figure 3. The anatomy of the brain

region to scan, demanding expensive equipment and experienced technicians. Using CT, MRI and SPECT scans (see pages 11–13), Professor Smith's group and others have proven that there is increasing damage in this region. This is also where there are more neurofibrillary tangles and beta-amyloid plaques – the hallmarks of Alzheimer's. These indicate damage and chaos to the normal network of neurons and their connections.

Since information is passed from and to the medial temporal lobe from other parts of the brain, as this area becomes more damaged, fewer signals are sent to other parts of the brain. These then also start to decline, becoming more and more disconnected, with ever-decreasing blood flow. The diagram on the following page shows the likely scenario. You'll notice that the beginning of damage is estimated to occur as early as 40 years before a person is diagnosed with dementia. That is why the message of this book is to start your prevention plan young.

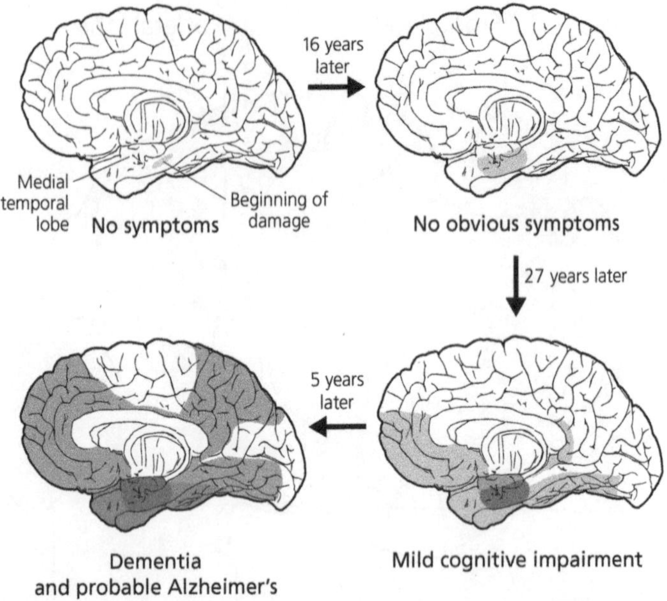

Figure 4. Progression of damage seen in Alzheimer's disease. In the top left diagram we see the first evidence of damage to the medial temporal lobe. This becomes easily visible in the second scan. By the third scan areas of the brain that connect to the medial temporal lobe are becoming increasingly damaged and cognitive impairment is diagnosed. In the fourth scan there is major damage to the medial temporal lobe and associated areas of the brain and a diagnosis of dementia. Taken from Smith A.D., 'Imaging the progression of Alzheimer pathology through the brain', *Proc Natl Acad Sci*, 99(7): 4135–37 (2002)

So far I've talked about the spread of damage seen in Alzheimer's, starting with the medial temporal lobe, and radiating out to other areas of the brain, which are in effect starved of signals, much as a muscle atrophies through lack of use. I've also mentioned other indicators of Alzheimer's such as neurofibrillary tangles, the lack of blood flow in the brain, the presence of beta-amyloid plaques, and, in the preceding chapter, the presence of high levels of homocysteine in the blood.

Exactly which of these factors 'causes' Alzheimer's, or kickstarts the process of damage, is the subject of much debate and ongoing research. We'll have to wait some years to find the answers.

Clues to curbing the epidemic

At the other end of the spectrum, scientists have been looking for ways to prevent Alzheimer's disease, and are conducting more and more studies revealing the specific dietary and lifestyle factors that greatly increase or decrease risk. For example, having a high intake of omega-3 fats and B vitamins appears to reduce risk, while consuming a lot of sugar and alcohol increases the risk.

Somewhere in the middle, scientists are discovering how changes in diet could cause changes in the brain. An example of this is the discovery of an enzyme that both regulates insulin – the key hormone for keeping your blood sugar in balance – and beta-amyloid. In a study published in the *Proceedings of the National Academy of Science*, mice modified to lack the enzyme insulysin, which breaks down insulin, had brain levels of beta-amyloid 1.5 times greater than those of normal mice.[14]

Researchers at the University of Washington School of Medicine in Seattle have also discovered a relationship between the development of Alzheimer's disease and disturbances in insulin and glucose metabolism, possibly explaining why people with diabetes have a much higher risk of developing Alzheimer's disease.[15] (Note that in Chapters 13 and 14, I go into why sugar and stress are your brain's worse enemies.)

However, the most exciting discovery is the role of B vitamins and how too little can lead to increases in homocysteine in the blood. Since neither beta-amyloid nor those neurofibrillary tangles can be measured before its too late, the discovery that levels of a simple chemical in your blood, easily gauged by a home-test kit, could be the best predictor of all is the most welcome news – and it should, in my opinion, revolutionise the early diagnosis and preventative treatment of those most likely to develop Alzheimer's.

In Chapter 7 I'll be discussing the results of two recent trials that report that supplementing high doses of specific B vitamins, designed to lower homocysteine levels, has the power to arrest age-related memory decline and substantially slow down Alzheimer's in the early stages, though sadly not in the moderately severe stage.

Working towards a happy ending

In the final stages of Alzheimer's, the sufferer completely loses touch with their surroundings and the ability to interact with others. Other complications can include bedsores, broken bones, increased susceptibility to infections and incontinence. It's not pretty. On average, the length of time between diagnosis and death is 6 to 8 years, but it may range from under 2 years to over 20.

Needless to say, this condition is traumatic for both sufferers and their friends and families, so the widespread ignorance about Alzheimer's preventability is little short of a tragedy.

It is likely that most people who get a diagnosis of probable Alzheimer's start to show the first signs of degeneration 10 years earlier, and possibly the first signs of brain changes 20 years earlier. So it's vital to act early. The key to prevention is to understand the contributing factors and to do something about them as soon as possible. Right now, because the thought of Alzheimer's is so terrifying, most people avoid even seeing their doctor and are usually diagnosed only in the late stages, usually reported by a relative who has found their partner becoming unmanageable. I hope this book, and the substantiated hope it provides, will encourage more people to seek help for age-related memory decline by putting into action the simple prevention steps summarised in Part 2.

4

How to Assess and Reverse Your Risk

WE'VE NOW SEEN HOW complex Alzheimer's is, and how this disease has no single cause. Many researchers are now beginning to agree on the idea that it is a degenerative disease that develops largely due to the long-term consequence of faulty nutrition and exposure to anti-nutrients, much like cardiovascular disease, and that multiple factors have to be in place for the condition to develop.

My aim for you is to make sure you know what these factors are so you can reduce your total risk. Since the majority are related to what you put in your mouth, any long-term solution must involve fundamental changes to your diet.

The contributory factors include:

- A genetic predisposition
- Inflammation
- Lack of antioxidant nutrients
- Lack of omega-3 fatty acids

- Excessive stress and elevated cortisol
- Raised homocysteine
- Lack of B vitamins
- Indigestion and/or malabsorption
- Poor liver detoxification
- Possibly excess aluminium, copper or mercury
- Acetylcholine and precursor deficiency
- Serotonin and precursor deficiency
- Dopamine and precursor deficiency
- Poor circulation.

Aside from a genetic predisposition, each of these can be prevented, as I will show you in Part 2 – and these prevention steps go to form the basis of my Alzheimer's Prevention Diet. But be aware that having the genetic predisposition on its own is not enough to cause the disease. Let me explain.

Not all in the genes

There is a great deal of hype about the role of genes in causing disease. Genes contain the instructions for building protein in the body and brain. Some proteins are used for building things like cells, in which case a faulty gene could mean a faulty building material. Many proteins are used to build enzymes. Enzymes do the work of the body, turning one substance into another. Down's syndrome – which involves an excess of a set of genes – is one example of a genetic condition where enzymes are out of kilter. What happens is that various enzymes needed to protect the body from oxidants don't work correctly and, as a consequence, someone with Down's syndrome experiences more rapid degeneration of their brain and body.

Since enzymes also depend on specific nutrients called co-factors or co-enzymes, supplying these in optimal amounts can make faulty enzyme systems work much better. Some children with Down's syndrome have made massive improvements in intelligence when treated with such a tailor-made 'optimum nutrition' approach.[16]

Very rare forms of Alzheimer's disease are due to mutations in one of three different genes. These are the so-called familial cases, where the onset of the disease is always seen before the age of 65, and they account for 1 per cent of all cases.

Many studies looking at the commonest form of late-onset Alzheimer's have focused on a gene called apolipoprotein E, or ApoE for short. It provides the instructions for transporting cholesterol and building healthy membranes for the brain's neurons. Those who inherit a particular type of this gene, called ApoE4, have more than double the risk of developing Alzheimer's, probably because the abnormal membrane building it causes results in too many beta-amyloid plaques. The presence of this defective gene is now being used as a marker to predict risk.

However, it's not just the presence of this gene that is important, but whether it is activated or 'expressed', to use the medical jargon. Think of your genes as software. It's not whether you have the software that counts. It's whether that program is currently running on your computer. Similarly, if you are one of the 25 per cent of the population that has the ApoE4 gene mutation, this will only increase your risk if this gene is activated and/or if other risk factors are also present.[17] So there are plenty of elderly people who carry the ApoE4 gene, but never develop Alzheimer's.

Recently three more contributor genes were discovered, called CLU and PICALM and CR1.[18] What's interesting is that most of these genes are involved in inflammatory processes. This implies that Alzheimer's may be another inflammatory disease and the brain damage may be a consequence of such inflammation.

The hot area of research is what activates ApoE4. Two current candidates are infection and faulty nutrition. Viruses, for example, can damage genes and change the message they deliver to brain cells, causing cellular damage. The question then becomes: what protects your genes from such damage? The answer may be enhanced methylation (that means lowering your homocysteine level) and improved antioxidation, which means eating more fruit and veg, as well as supplementing key antioxidant nutrients such as vitamins A, C and E.

Another gene that may be involved is one that's necessary for keeping your homocysteine level low. It has the memorable name of the MTHFR 677C>T, and contains the instructions for building an enzyme called methylenetetrahydrofolate reductase. Try saying that! (Don't worry – it's called MTHFR for short.) MTHFR helps convert toxic homocysteine into the harmless and brain-friendly amino acid SAMe. Approximately 1 in 10 people have this genetic difference and consequently are more prone to having higher homocysteine levels, which means a greater risk for Alzheimer's disease and memory problems later in life. Your likelihood of having it is highest if you are Mexican (32 per cent have it) or Italian, especially from Sicily or Campania (20 per cent have it), and lowest if you are of African (2 per cent) or Asian (3.8 per cent) origin.[19]

Even if you do have this condition, you can do something about it. The solution is simple if you know how. You can improve how well your enzymes work by increasing your intake of the right co-enzymes or co-factors – in this particular case vitamins B2, B6, B12, folic acid and TMG.

An inflammatory issue?

It is highly likely that both cardiovascular disease and Alzheimer's result at least in part from the same or a similar disease process. In cardiovascular disease the arteries become inflamed and damaged. A similar process occurs in the brain in Alzheimer's disease. Often, the two diseases occur together. A review carried out at New York University's neurology department highlights the fact that at least a third of patients with Alzheimer's also have some degree of vascular disease. Not only does the presence of cardiovascular disease greatly increase the chances of getting Alzheimer's, especially if you have the ApoE4 gene,[20] but many causative factors apply to both conditions.

It's one of those chicken or egg situations. For example, having vascular disease tends to speed up the memory loss associated with Alzheimer's. Once cardiovascular disease is present, blockages in arteries may lead to a poor supply of key nutrients to the brain – a condition known as cerebrovascular disease. And without a good supply of antioxidants, brain cells become more vulnerable to damage from free radicals, rogue molecules produced by combustion, for example from frying foods or smoking. So cerebrovascular disease is intimately linked to both a lack of antioxidants and excess exposure to oxidants. Antioxidant nutrients such as vitamins C and E have been shown to help both conditions – not only to mop up these brain pollutants, but also to reduce inflammation.

Cerebrovascular disease is also strongly linked to having a high homocysteine level. Based on an analysis of all current research, having a high homocysteine level makes you more than twice as likely to develop Alzheimer's as having cerebrovascular disease. A high H score also makes you much more likely to develop cerebrovascular disease. So, whichever way you cut it, keeping your homocysteine level low is essential.

All of these factors – a lack of antioxidants, too many brain pollutants, the presence of cardiovascular or cerebrovascular disease – tend to increase the risk and severity of Alzheimer's, with the critical link being inflammation. Now, let's explore how this inflammation occurs, and how to prevent it.

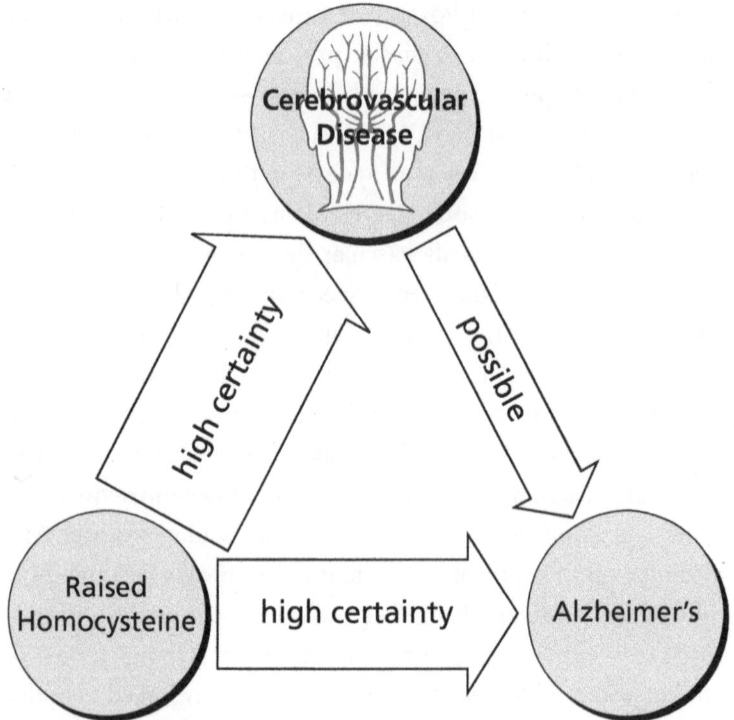

Figure 5. Cerebrovascular disease, homocysteine and Alzheimer's disease risk. The studies to date show that there is a high certainty that raised homocysteine is causally linked to Alzheimer's disease, while only a possibility that cerebrovascular disease is causally linked to Alzheimer's

We've seen how the presence of beta-amyloid plaques or remains of dead cells and other waste material in the brain distinguish Alzheimer's from other forms of dementia. Beta-amyloid is an abnormal protein that is also found in the plaques of arterial deposits. It is a toxic invader that arises when the body is in 'emergency mode', as can happen when a person's total environmental overload exceeds their genetic capacity to adapt. In such cases, the person's immune system can become overreactive and trigger inflammation.

In fact, most major diseases involve inflammation. That includes cardiovascular disease, as we've seen, diabetes, cancer, and any that end in 'itis' – colitis, arthritis, bronchitis and sinusitis, for instance.

So, looked at in this way, the presence of the ApoE4 gene simply means a person has less genetic capacity to adapt to the insults of today's diets and lifestyles. But this weakness can be countered by optimum nutrition, which endows us with more adaptive capacity by giving the brain and body a less toxic chemical environment. Inflammation, in this model, is the alarm bell. It's your body telling you something is wrong.

To get rid of inflammation you have to get to the root cause, and we'll be finding out how digestive problems, too much sugar and stress, a lack of antioxidants and too much homocysteine can all lead to inflammation.

Looking at Alzheimer's as an inflammatory disease also explains why taking anti-inflammatory drugs offers some protection from it, which is consistent with the hypothesis that the damage that occurs to brain cells is part of an overall inflammatory reaction. But, as you can see in the diagram overleaf, many of these drugs end up encouraging inflammation in the long run by damaging the gut, which leads to more inflammation!

Luckily, there are natural anti-inflammatory nutrients that don't harm the digestive tract, and these may prove to be more effective, both in the long run and in preventing inflammation – especially as cortisone-based anti-inflammatory drugs may make matters worse. Antioxidants and omega-3 fats are effective anti-inflammatories. There are also some very powerful anti-inflammatory herbs, such as turmeric (the well-known yellow curry spice), which I'll be recommending in Chapter 16.

We've been through a number of risk factors for developing Alzheimer's. You can check out your own risk of developing Alzheimer's or dementia in the Alzheimer's Risk Factors Check on page 38.

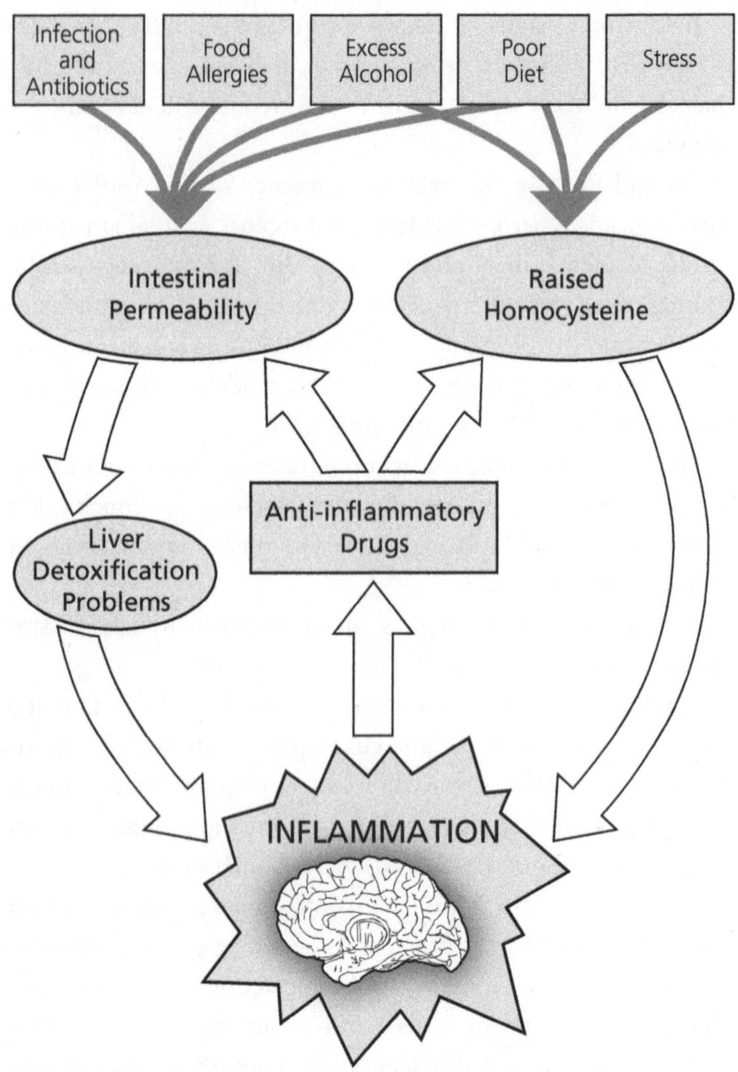

Figure 6. How what you eat leads to inflammation. Excess alcohol, stress and poor diet raise homocysteine, which promotes inflammation in the brain. Gut infections, antibiotics, food allergies, excess alcohol and poor diet increase intestinal permeability, which overloads the liver, leading to inflammation in the brain. Anti-inflammatory drugs lessen inflammation, but can increase intestinal permeability and homocysteine, thus making matters worse in the long-run

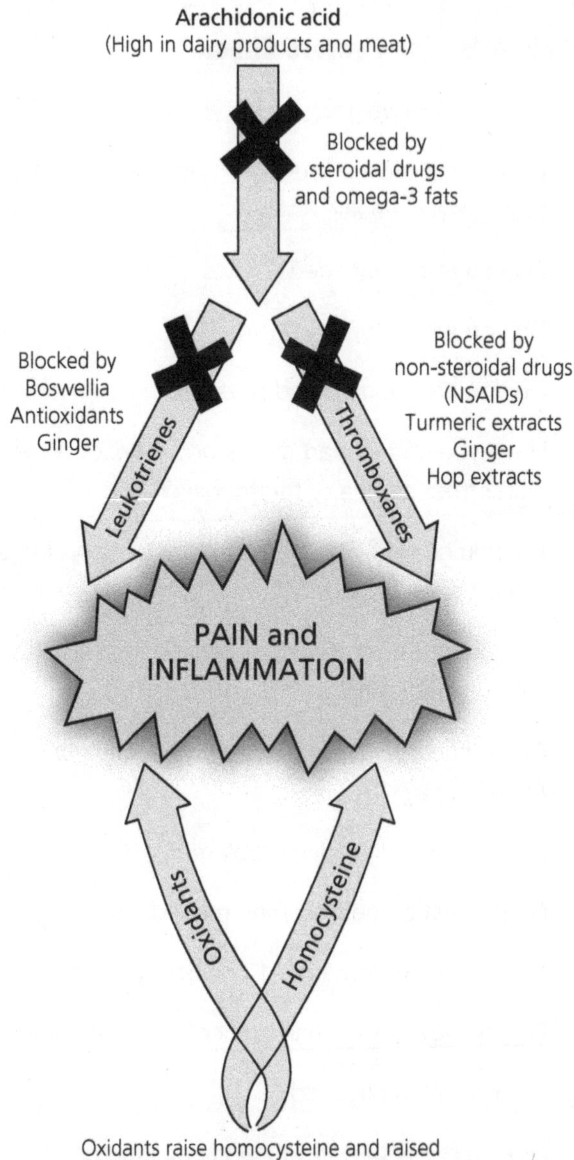

Figure 7. A diet high in antioxidants and homocysteine-lowering B vitamins, and low in meat and dairy products and high in omega-3 fats, together with plenty of ginger, turmeric and anti-inflammatory herbs including boswellia and hop extracts, helps to reduce inflammation and pain

Alzheimer's Risk Factors Check

- [ ] Are you overweight?
- [ ] Do you eat oily fish such as mackerel or sardines less than once a week?
- [ ] Do you rarely eat seeds?
- [ ] Do you smoke?
- [ ] Do you have high blood pressure?
- [ ] Have you had a heart attack or stroke, or do you suffer from angina or thrombosis?
- [ ] Are you currently taking anti-inflammatory drugs such as cortisone or NSAIDS?
- [ ] Do you eat fewer than four servings of fruit and vegetables a day?
- [ ] Do you have a family history of dementia or Alzheimer's?
- [ ] Do you have digestive problems?
- [ ] Do you eat something fried most days?
- [ ] Do you drink more than 10 units of alcohol a week?
- [ ] Do you have more than one coffee or tea every day?
- [ ] Are you often stressed?
- [ ] Do you rarely take B vitamin supplements?
- [ ] Do you rarely take antioxidant supplements, including vitamins C and E?

- ☐ If you've had a homocysteine test, was your score above 10?
- ☐ If you've had a homocysteine test, was your score above 15?
- ☐ Is your score on the Mind and Memory Check (page 8) more than 4?
- ☐ Is your score on the Mind and Memory Check more than 6?

If you gave more than 6 'yes' answers you have probably increased your risk by half.

If you gave more than 12 'yes' answers you may have doubled your risk.

If you gave more than 16 'yes' answers you may have quadrupled your risk.

But don't worry. Instead, put your energy into turning all 'yes' answers into 'no's by making simple changes to your diet and lifestyle. Now fill in your scores on Your Brain's MOT chart, in Appendix 1, page 205. I'll tell you how to use this information to build your own personalised Alzheimer's Prevention Plan in Part 3.

5

Neuroanalysis – How to Tune Up Your Brain

YOUR BRAIN SINGS TO the tune of some 40 neurotransmitters, but five of them are particularly relevant to our memory and moods. These are the chemicals that deliver messages between your brain cells and have the ability to make you deliriously happy or dangerously crazy, sharp as a razor or completely forgetful, relaxed or anxious. The balance between these neurotransmitters in your brain has a profound effect on how you think, feel and act.

Let's meet these influential players in the field of mind, memory and mood.

ACETYLCHOLINE is the 'brainy' neurotransmitter and is associated with thought, memory and learning. Levels are high during waking consciousness and also during dreaming. However, they are low during deep sleep. Levels are also low in adults suffering from memory decline and dementia and in some children with attention deficit disorder. Acetylcholine is made from the nutrient choline, which is abundant in eggs and fish.

(An enzyme dependent on pantothenic acid or vitamin B5 adds on the acetyl part.)

SEROTONIN is the 'happy' neurotransmitter because your level of it has a profound influence on your mood. Without enough, you can end up feeling flat and depressed. Levels tend to rise in the evening, but the brain stops releasing it when you dream. It's made from the amino acid tryptophan. An enzyme dependent on vitamin B6 and zinc then converts it into 5–hydroxytryptophan (5–HTP) and then into serotonin. Alternatively, it can be turned into DMT (dimethyl tryptamine), a neurotransmitter-like chemical thought to be produced in the pineal gland. Serotonin itself can be turned into melatonin, a neurotransmitter produced in the pineal gland and released during sleep. Melatonin not only promotes healthy sleep, it also acts as an antioxidant, helping to repair the brain while you snooze.

DOPAMINE/ADRENALIN/NORADRENALIN are the 'motivators', giving you a zest for life. They are associated with the waking state. This trio, all produced from dopamine, keep you motivated, enthusiastic and up for living life to the full. Just about anything that makes you feel good – sex, being in love, dancing, music, coffee – is associated with a boost in the release of these neurotransmitters.

While dopamine and noradrenalin make up the feelgood factor, adrenalin is more associated with stress and 'get up and go'. If you don't have enough adrenalin, you've got no kickstart and can't deal with the stresses of life. If you don't have enough dopamine or noradrenalin, you don't feel good – you have little enthusiasm for life.

These three neurotransmitters are made from the amino acids L-phenylalanine (DLPA) and tyrosine. These turn into dopamine first, then noradrenalin, then adrenalin. The enzymes needed to do this depend on B vitamins, especially B6, folic acid, B12 and niacin.

GLUTAMATE is an amino acid and an 'excitatory' neurotransmitter that stimulates nerve cells to fire. It is particularly important in the laying down of memories and in the communication between neurons in different parts of the cerebral cortex. It is the glutamate-using neurons that die in the medial temporal lobe in Alzheimer's disease. These glutamate-using neurons can be fine-tuned by the other neurotransmitters, especially GABA (see below) and acetylcholine.

GABA, short for gamma-amino-butyric acid, is the 'cool' neurotransmitter, relaxing and calming you down after a burst of adrenalin. If adrenalin is the accelerator, GABA is the brakes. It's made from an amino acid called glutamate and is also associated with memory, keeping you calm and clear-headed. It appears to facilitate the recording of memories into cells. Glutamate is an amino acid and is also made from L-glutamine. GABA and glutamate are both part of the same family, one being 'excitatory' and the other 'inhibitory'.

Most people show deficiencies and imbalances in these five neurotransmitters as they start to experience a loss of mental acuity and concentration, motivation or mood. There are four reasons why you might be short of any one of these neurotransmitters:

1. First, you might be deficient in the materials from which they are made. These are specific amino acids found in protein, plus certain vitamins and minerals needed to assemble these building blocks into neurotransmitters.
2. Secondly, you may be a poor 'builder'. For example, if you have a high homocysteine level and are therefore poor at methylation, you won't build your neurotransmitters so efficiently.

3. Thirdly, your lifestyle and the way you react to things may be creating an excessive demand. For example, if you are stressed out and working long hours in a demanding job you can literally overtax your adrenal system, leaving you less able to cope with stress when you need to. Similarly, the see-saw of emotions in a tumultuous love affair, or an unresolvable crisis, can leave you burnt out.
4. Finally, since most neurotransmitters are produced in the brain, if your neurons are starting to die off, you make less of them.

So in people with Alzheimer's or other forms of dementia, having low levels of these neurotransmitters is extremely common.

Test your neurotransmitter balance

There are two ways to test your own neurotransmitter levels. The first, which you can do right now, is by checking yourself out on the questions overleaf. The second is by having a Neurotransmitter Profile blood test. More on this on page 50, but for now, I'd like you to answer the following questions, scoring one point for each 'yes' answer.

DIY neurotransmitter testing

Acetylcholine Check

- [ ] Do you lack imagination?
- [ ] Do you have difficulty remembering names when you first meet people?
- [ ] Have you noticed that your memory ability is decreasing?
- [ ] Have you been accused of being unromantic?
- [ ] Do you have difficulty remembering friends' birthdays?
- [ ] Do you feel you have lost some of your creativity?
- [ ] Do you suffer from insomnia?
- [ ] Have you lost muscle tone?
- [ ] Do you rarely exercise?
- [ ] Do you crave fatty foods?
- [ ] Have you consumed a fair amount of hallucinogens or other mind-altering drugs in the past?
- [ ] Do you rarely remember your dreams?
- [ ] Do you sometimes find it difficult to breathe?
- [ ] Add up your TOTAL SCORE (yes = 1 point)

Serotonin Check

- [ ] Do you think of yourself as not very perceptive?
- [ ] Do you have difficulty remembering things you've seen in the past?

- [ ] Do you have a slow reaction time?
- [ ] Do you have a poor sense of direction?
- [ ] Do you suffer from insomnia?
- [ ] Do you always wake up early in the morning?
- [ ] Do you find it hard to relax?
- [ ] Do you wake up at least two times during the night?
- [ ] Do you find it hard to fall asleep when you've been awakened?
- [ ] Are you often sad?
- [ ] Are you easily irritated?
- [ ] Do you have thoughts of self-destruction?
- [ ] Have you had suicidal thoughts at times in your life?

[ ] TOTAL SCORE

Dopamine Check

- [ ] Do you have trouble paying consistent attention and concentrating?
- [ ] Do you need caffeine to wake up?
- [ ] Do you have difficulty thinking quickly enough?
- [ ] Do you have a poor attention span?
- [ ] Do you have trouble getting through a task even when it is interesting?
- [ ] Do you crave sugar?
- [ ] Do you have decreased libido?

cont. overleaf

- [ ] Do you sleep too much?
- [ ] Do you have a history of alcohol overuse or addiction?
- [ ] Do you often feel exhausted for no apparent reason?
- [ ] Has maintaining your weight been a constant struggle?
- [ ] Do you have trouble getting out of bed in the morning?
- [ ] Do you have cravings for, or have you ever been addicted to, caffeine, cocaine, amphetamines or ecstasy?

[ ] TOTAL SCORE

GABA Check

- [ ] Do you have difficulty remembering phone numbers?
- [ ] Do you have trouble finding the right word?
- [ ] Does your ability to focus come and go?
- [ ] When you read, do you have to go back over the same paragraph a few times to absorb the information?
- [ ] Do you sometimes feel shaky?
- [ ] Do you sometimes tremble?
- [ ] Do you have frequent backaches and/or headaches?
- [ ] Do you sometimes get short of breath?
- [ ] Do you tend to have cold hands?
- [ ] Are you sometimes dizzy?
- [ ] Do you often have muscle tension?

- [ ] Are you often nervous and/or do you get butterflies in your stomach?
- [ ] Do you often feel tired even when you have had a good night's sleep?
- [ ] TOTAL SCORE

If you answered 'yes' more than eight times within any one section, the chances are that you have some level of deficiency in this particular neurotransmitter. Now fill in your scores on Your Brain's MOT chart, in Appendix 1 on page 205.

If you suspect you're deficient...

ACETYLCHOLINE A deficiency in this neurotransmitter makes it likely that your memory and imagination will be deteriorating. You'll dream less, and be more confused, forgetful, disoriented and disorganised as you lose your mental traction.

The following foods, drinks, drugs and activities are bad news for you:

Sugar, deep-fried food, junk and refined food, smoking, alcohol (except for the odd occasion), passively watching television.

The following habits will be especially good for you:

Learning new things, engaging in stimulating conversations, outdoor exercise, planning your day and making a daily 'to do' list, establishing a daily routine, taking your supplements every day.

The following foods will be especially good for you:

Organic/free range eggs and fish, especially salmon (aim for wild or organic rather than farmed), mackerel, sardines and tuna.

The following supplements will be especially good for you:

Lecithin, phosphatidyl choline, phosphatidyl serine, DMAE, pantothenic acid (vitamin B5), DHA/EPA (omega-3s).

SEROTONIN If you are serotonin deficient, you are likely to have a low mood and difficulty sleeping. You are more likely to feel 'disconnected'. You may not feel much love for life or joie de vivre.

The following foods, drinks, drugs and activities are bad news for you:

Alcohol, sleeping pills, late nights, excessive solitude.

Developing the following habits will be especially good for you:

Dancing to music, seeing people, having a massage, exploring new relationships, long walks in nature, watching the sunset or sunrise, getting a pet or looking after someone else's, playing with children, playing games, travelling to somewhere exotic or unusual, exploring new cultures, doing what you enjoy the most.

The following foods will be especially good for you:

Fish, fruit as snacks, eggs, avocado, wheatgerm, low-fat cheese, chicken, turkey and duck.

The following supplements will be especially good for you:

Tryptophan, 5–hydroxytryptophan (5–HTP), vitamin B6, magnesium, zinc.

DOPAMINE If you are currently dopamine deficient, you will lack drive, motivation, enthusiasm and get up and go. You will also crave stimulants, especially caffeine, to give you a kickstart.

The following foods, drinks, drugs and activities are bad news for you:

Strong tea, coffee, caffeinated drinks, caffeine pills (ProPlus), guarana, amphetamines, cocaine, gambling, high-risk activities and adventures, lack of sleep, excessive exercise, rocky relationships.

Developing the following habits will be especially good for you:

Getting enough sleep but not too much, establishing a routine, exercise in the morning, regular meals, delegation, meditation, yoga, t'ai chi, artistic pursuits.

The following supplements will help you restore your balance:

Tyrosine, phenylalanine, DHEA (in the short term only), B vitamins, vitamin C (1 to 4 grams, spread out through the day).

GABA If you are GABA deficient you'll find it hard to relax. You can't switch off and live in a state of permanent anxiety, always worried about something and on edge, with bursts of anger, irritability and self-criticism.

The following foods, drinks, drugs and activities are bad news for you:

Sugar, alcohol, benzodiazepines (e.g. Valium), sleeping pills, cannabis, because they 'down-regulate' your brain to the calming effects of GABA. Also avoid stressors such as strong tea, coffee, caffeinated drinks, caffeine pills (ProPlus), guarana, amphetamines, gambling, high-risk activities and adventures, lack of sleep, excessive exercise, rocky relationships.

Developing the following habits will be especially good for you:

Meditation, reading fiction, artistic endeavours, beach holidays.

The following foods will be especially good for you:

Broccoli, spinach and anything green – the darker the better – plus seeds and nuts, potatoes, bananas, citrus fruit, eggs.

The following supplements will be especially good for you:

Glutamine, glutamic acid, taurine, inositol, magnesium.

The Neurotransmitter Profile blood test

We've seen how it's possible to gauge a probable deficiency in a particular neurotransmitter by examining how we feel in detail. But you might be wondering whether you can accurately test your level and balance of these important neurotransmitters. The answer is yes. However, it's not a straightforward process. Since the brain is bathed in a fluid called the cerebrospinal fluid, or CSF for short, measuring neurotransmitter levels in the CSF would probably be the most accurate method. However, this would involve a lumbar puncture – a procedure that's far too invasive to recommend.

Overall blood or urine levels of neurotransmitters seem to bear little relation to the levels in CSF. Some scientists have also tried to deduce what's going on in the brain by looking for the breakdown products of neurotransmitters in the blood or urine. Again, this is far from accurate.

What is proving most accurate and useful is the level of some neurotransmitters in what are called the 'platelets' in the blood. These are tiny disk-shaped structures whose function is mostly related to the clotting of blood after injury. The amounts of neurotransmitters within the platelets are very low, so incredibly sensitive measurement techniques are needed.

Heading this research is Professor Tapan Audhya from New York University Medical Center, whose Vitamin Diagnostics laboratory is now making such tests available. Audhya's research has shown that while serotonin levels in blood or urine bear no resemblance to CSF levels, the serotonin platelet levels reflect CSF levels quite accurately.[21] He has also proven that when you give a person the necessary amino acids, for example 5–HTP, that the brain needs to restore normal levels of serotonin, platelet levels and CSF levels also go up.[22]

While neurotransmitter testing is in its infancy, at the Brain Bio Centre in London – a nutritional treatment centre for mental health, where I am clinical director – we measure the platelet levels of some of these neurotransmitters and then adjust a person's diet and supplementation accordingly. (See Resources, page 248, for details on the Brain Bio Centre as well as these and other tests.) To discover more about the testing process at the Brain Bio Centre, see the case study overleaf.

Case study

John came to the Brain Bio Centre complaining of problems with his memory, and difficulty concentrating. He and his family were very concerned about his condition and wanted to do all they could to preserve his memory.

In addition to reviewing his diet, we ran a number of tests including those checking neurotransmitter status. The results showed that his levels of all the neurotransmitters tested were low, as were some key nutrients, such as zinc and magnesium. Within a few months of an improved diet and a comprehensive nutritional supplement programme, John came to see us again and was very happy to report that he was feeling much more mentally alert and wasn't struggling so much with his memory.

Balancing the brain's neurotransmitter activity

We've looked at each neurotransmitter in isolation. But at the very start of this chapter I talked about how a balance between them is vital in keeping your brain in tune. Let's look in more detail at how this works.

The balance of neurotransmitter activity in your brain reflects shifts in your state from awake to asleep, relaxed to alert, focused to daydreaming. This pattern of activity can also be measured as brain waves. Each pattern results in a certain type of electrical activity, from the very fast 'beta' waves, consistent with being awake and alert, to the very slow 'delta' waves that occur in deep sleep. When you are relaxed, you have more 'alpha' wave activity; and when you are either dreaming or in a more connected state, for example in deep meditation or during a burst of artistic creativity, you have more 'theta' wave activity.

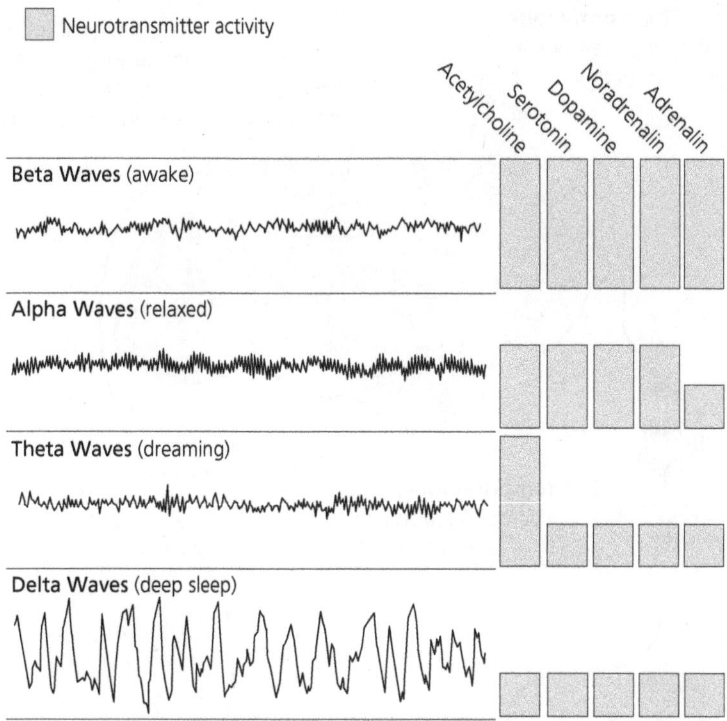

Figure 8. When you are awake there is much more neurotransmitter activity than when you are in deep sleep. When you dream, acetylcholine activity is high

Each of these different brain wave patterns is associated with certain parts of the brain. For example, the beta waves that occur when you're awake and alert are located mainly in the frontal lobes of the brain. These lobes are vital for your working memory, and initiating actions.

The parietal lobe, which sits behind the frontal lobe and on top of the temporal lobes, is associated more with alpha waves and with processing sensory information that comes into the brain, helping the brain understand and make sense of the world. In a way, this part of the brain gives you an immediate memory of identifying sensory information.

The temporal lobes, below the parietal lobes, are vital for

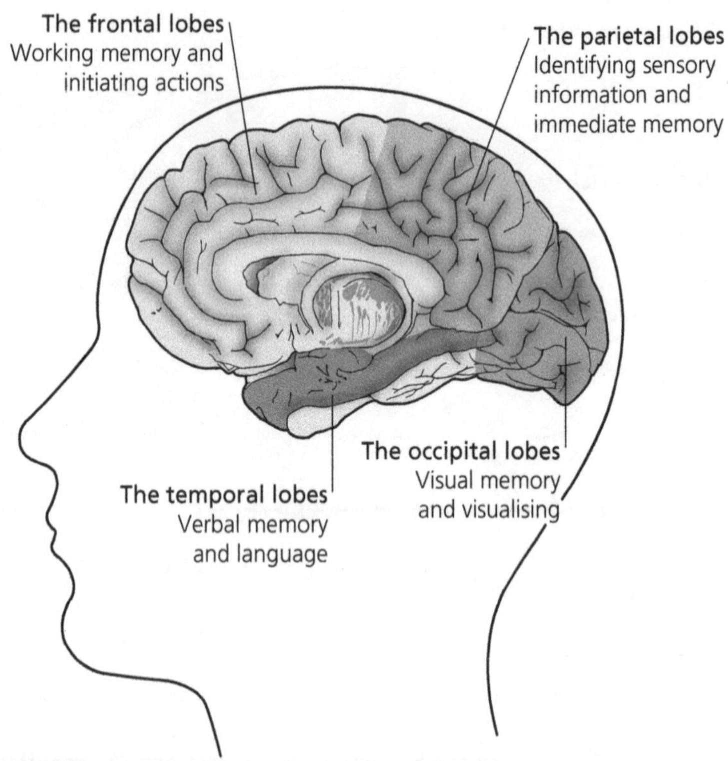

Figure 9. The relationship between the lobes of the brain and different functions

memory and language, and hence are the home of verbal memories.

The occipital lobes, at the rear of the brain, are very important for visual memory, and for visualising.

Restoring the rhythm of your brain

When your neurotransmitter balance and your brain wave pattern are out of kilter, you feel it. But how you cope with it makes all the difference between brain health and a slide into serious problems.

Self-medicating

Many of us self-medicate unknowingly by eating, drinking or smoking substances that temporarily promote the neurotransmitter we lack. Caffeine is a good example. Caffeine causes a short-term boost to your adrenalin levels, giving you some drive and motivation. Nicotine triggers the release of dopamine, GABA, glutamate, adrenalin and acetylcholine, while dampening the effect of serotonin. Sugar can also increase amounts of dopamine in the short term.

But all of these substances are – unsurprisingly – bad news in the long term. They blunt your brain and make it progressively less sensitive to its own neurotransmitters and less able to produce healthy patterns of brain wave activity, a process called down-regulation. It happens because substances like coffee block the enzyme that would normally break down excessive adrenalin, hence your adrenalin levels can soar five times higher after coffee. This is like turning up the volume too high in your brain, forcing the brain to protect itself by blocking its 'neurotransmitter ears', which are the receptor sites for adrenalin. The more often you do this, the deafer your brain becomes and the more of the stimulant you need to get going. This is why these substances are addictive.

Pharmaceutical drugs

The pharmaceutical industry cottoned on to this dynamic many years ago and has produced a number of drugs that block the breakdown of neurotransmitters or interfere with their actions. Valium and other benzodiazepines promote the action of GABA, so you relax and stop feeling anxious. Long term, however, you become increasingly insensitive to your own GABA and can't relax without taking a tranquilliser. In short, you're addicted.

More recent drugs, such as 'selective serotonin reuptake

Normally we release enough neurotransmitters to feel good. But not too many to cause down-regulation.

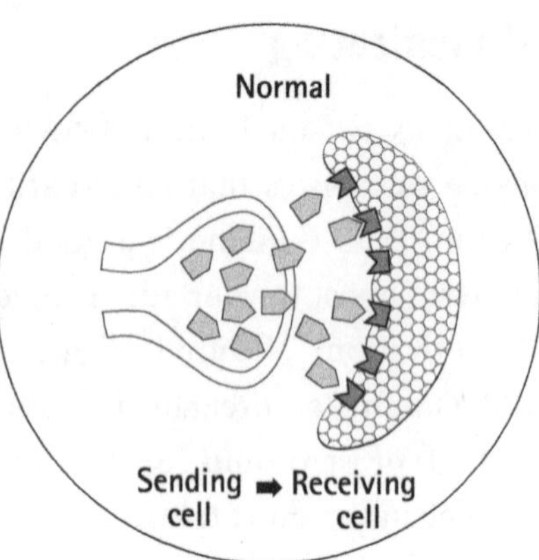

Over-stimulation, which is what many drugs do, leads to too many neurotransmitters being released. The body fights back by shutting down receptor sites, making you more tolerant to drugs and stimulants, which is why you crave more.

Down-regulation
More neurotransmitters fewer receptors

Sending ➡ Receiving
cell cell

If you quit stimulants or drugs, to begin with you feel low because you don't have enough neurotransmitters. The body helps you recover by opening up more receptor sites, making you more sensitive to your body's own neurotransmitters.

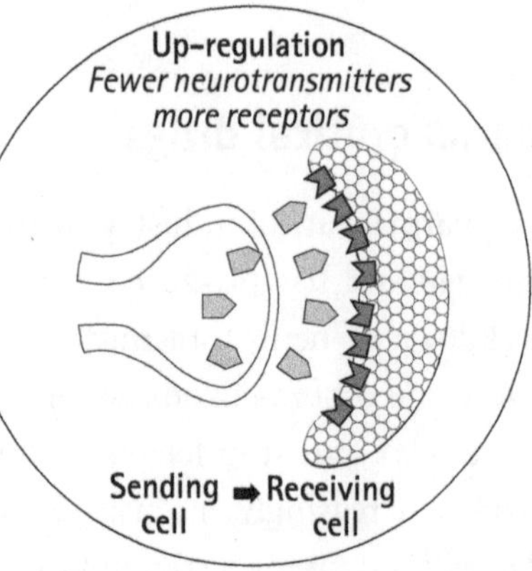

Figure 10. Down-regulation

inhibitor' antidepressants (Prozac, sertraline, paroxetine and Lustral, to name a few) work in a similar, but slightly different way. Instead of blocking the breakdown of serotonin, they block its reuptake. In simple language this means that the brain recycles its neurotransmitters after releasing them into the synapse between brain cells, to use them again. If you block their re-uptake you get a temporary boost to your serotonin status. But at what cost in the future?

It is well known that people often feel worse when they try to stop taking these drugs. These used to be called 'cessation' effects, but the British government has asked drug companies to come clean and call them what they are – withdrawal effects. It is highly likely that these drugs, too, are addictive.

The most commonly prescribed drugs for Alzheimer's and other forms of dementia are acetylcholinesterase inhibitors such as Aricept. These stop the brain from breaking down acetyl-choline, the memory transmitter. These drugs don't deal with the underlying causes of the neuronal damage. What they do is boost the brain's levels of this neurotransmitter.

Increased concentrations of acetylcholine lead to increased communication between nerve cells, which may in turn temporarily improve or stabilise the symptoms of Alzheimer's disease. This produces improvement in about 20 per cent of people with Alzheimer's, but only as long as there are enough neurons. So, as the disease progresses, the drugs rapidly stop working, although they don't appear to change the progression of the underlying disease process in any way.

The longest ever trial of Aricept in people with Alzheimer's took place over four years. Published in the *Lancet* in 2004, this study found no difference in 'worthwhile improvements' – such as rates of disease progression, the rate at which people were placed in nursing homes, caregiver time, or behaviour decline – regardless of the dosage given.[23] However, during the first two years of the study, patients taking Aricept (some participants were given a placebo) did do slightly better in tests gauging thinking and functional ability. But Richard Gray, the study's lead researcher, concluded, 'Realistically, patients are unlikely to derive much benefit from this drug.'

Moreover, there are some unpleasant side-effects with acetylcholinerstase inhibitors, including nausea and vomiting, diarrhoea, stomach cramps and headaches, dizziness, fatigue, insomnia and loss of appetite.

Restoration with nutrients

If drugs, from caffeine to Prozac, aren't the long-term solution to restoring neurotransmitter balance, what is? We've already seen the answer. It's to give your brain all the nutrients it needs to make its own neurotransmitters. This means taking vitamins, minerals, amino acids and also phospholipids, from which the brain can make acetylcholine.

The DIY approach is, admittedly, more work for you. It does mean changing your diet and taking supplements. However, the long-term results are far better, and there are virtually no side-effects, since the brain is well used to working with naturally occurring brain nutrients. They are not, after all, alien to your brain and body chemistry, nor are they toxic to the brain, even in amounts several times higher than I'll be recommending for you.

On the page opposite there is a handy recap of the information I provided earlier in this chapter.

In Part 3, I'll explain exactly how to build your own 'brain protection plan' based on your personalised scores in Your Brain's MOT (see page 205). This will involve a diet and a range of supplements. Many of these nutrients come in combination supplements so you won't need to take lots of individual capsules.

But first, let's look at the four absolutely essential brain nutrients that everybody needs, regardless of any individual imbalances. These I call the four essential brain foods. In the next chapter you can check out your current diet to know which brain foods you need to be eating on a regular basis.

The Key Neurotransmitter Nutrients

Acetylcholine	Phosphatidyl choline Phosphatidyl serine Pantothenic acid (B5) DHA/EPA (omega-3s)
Dopamine, Adrenalin, Noradrenalin	Phenylalanine Tyrosine Vitamin B12 Vitamin C
GABA	Glutamine Glutamic acid Taurine Inositol Magnesium
Serotonin	Tryptophan 5–HTP Vitamin B6 Magnesium Zinc

6

The Essential Brain Foods – Check Yourself Out

WHETHER YOU'RE IN good mental shape or are currently dealing with a declining memory, there are four essential foods you need to tune up your brain.

- Essential fats – these keep your brain 'well oiled'
- Phospholipids – these memory molecules give 'oomph' to the brain
- Amino acids – these are the brain's messengers
- Intelligent nutrients – these include vitamins and minerals that 'fine-tune' your mind.

We've already encountered all these in the preceding chapters; now let's see whether you're deficient in them.

You are not only what you eat – how well you think, feel and remember all depend on what you eat! You can check out whether you are getting enough of these essential fats using the Essential Fat Check.

Essential Fat Check

- ☐ Do you eat oily fish (trout, sardines, herring, mackerel, wild or organic salmon or fresh tuna) less than once a week?
- ☐ Do you eat seeds or their cold-pressed oils less than three times a week?
- ☐ Do you eat meat or dairy products most days?
- ☐ Do you eat processed or fried foods (ready meals, chips, crisps) three or more times a week?
- ☐ Do you have dry or rough skin or a tendency to eczema?
- ☐ Do you have a poor memory or difficulty concentrating?
- ☐ Do you suffer from PMS or breast tenderness?
- ☐ Do you suffer from water retention?
- ☐ Do you suffer from dry, watery or itchy eyes?
- ☐ Do you have inflammatory health problems such as arthritis?

If you have answered 'yes' to more than five questions, you are very likely deficient in essential fats. Check whether your diet contains enough seeds, seed oils and oily fish.

Ultimately, however, the most accurate gauge of whether you're getting enough essential fats is to have a blood test. This gives you a complete breakdown of all the essential fats in your system and what you're lacking. These tests are available through clinical nutritionists.

Good fats, bad fats

Conclusive research now clearly shows that the amount and type of fat consumed during foetal development, infancy, childhood, adolescence, adulthood, old age, and indeed every day of your life, has a profound effect on how you think and feel. The brain and nervous system are totally dependent on a family of fats. These include:

- Saturated and monounsaturated fat
- Cholesterol
- Omega-3 (polyunsaturated) fat – especially EPA and DHA
- Omega-6 (polyunsaturated) fat – especially GLA and AA.

The first two types can be made in the body. The omega fats, however, have to be topped up through diet – so these are the ones we'll discuss here.

If you have been overexposed to low-fat dieting and are fat-phobic, however, you should know that you're depriving yourself of essential, health-giving nutrients. The same is true if the fats you do eat are 'hard' fat, either from the saturated kind found in dairy products or meat, or damaged fats found in many cakes, biscuits and other processed foods, fried foods and some margarines. In fact, unless you go out of your way to eat the right kind of fat-rich foods, or supplement essential fats, the chances are you're missing out on optimal health. Most people in the West are overdosing on saturated 'killer' fats, and undernourished in the essential, healing fats.

I'll explain more about the incredible healing properties of these essential fats in Chapter 10, but for now, so you can get started on boosting your brain power, here are some general guidelines to ensure you get enough brain fats.

- Eat seeds and nuts – the best are flax, hemp, pumpkin, sunflower and sesame. You get more goodness out of them by grinding them first and sprinkling on cereal, soups and salads.
- Eat coldwater carnivorous, or oily, fish – a serving of herring, mackerel, or wild salmon two or three times a week provides a good source of omega-3 fats (fresh tuna is good, too, but limit it to three times a month).
- Use cold-pressed seed oils – either choose an oil blend or hemp oil for salad dressings and other cold uses, such as drizzling on vegetables instead of butter.
- Minimise your intake of fried food, processed food and saturated fat from meat and dairy products.
- Supplement fish oil for omega-3 fats and starflower or evening primrose oil for omega-6 fats.

Phospholipid Check

- [ ] Do you eat fish (especially sardines) less than once a week?
- [ ] Do you eat fewer than 3 eggs per week?
- [ ] Do you eat liver, soya/tofu or nuts less than three times a week?
- [ ] Do you take less than 5g of lecithin each day?
- [ ] Is your memory declining?
- [ ] Do you sometimes go looking for something and forget what it was you were looking for?
- [ ] Do you find it hard to do calculations in your head?

cont. overleaf

- [ ] Do you sometimes have difficulty concentrating?
- [ ] Do you have a tendency towards depression?
- [ ] Are you a 'slow learner'?

If you ticked five or more in the 'yes' column, the chances are you're not getting enough phospholipids.

Phospholipids are 'smart' fats, not only enhancing your mood, mind and mental performance, as do omega-3 fats, but also protecting against age-related memory decline and Alzheimer's disease. They are also the insulation experts, helping make up the myelin that sheathes all nerves and so promoting a smooth run for all the signals in the brain.

There are two main kinds of phospholipids – phosphatidyl choline and phosphatidyl serine. Supplementing phosphatidyl choline and phosphatidyl serine has some very positive benefits for your brain. Research on rats at Duke University Medical Center in the US demonstrated that giving choline during pregnancy creates the equivalent of superbrains in the offspring.

The researchers fed pregnant rats choline halfway through their pregnancy. The infant rats whose mothers were given choline had vastly superior brains with more neuronal connections, and consequently, improved learning ability and better memory recall, all of which persisted into old age. This research showed that giving choline helps restructure the brain for improved performance.

The positive effects of supplementing phosphatidyl serine are equally amazing. In one study, supplementing PS improved the subjects' memories to the level of people 12 years younger. Dr Thomas Crook from the Memory Assessment Clinic in Bethesda, Maryland, gave 149 people with age-associated memory impairment a daily dose of 300mg of PS or a placebo. When tested after

12 weeks, the ability of those taking PS to match names to faces (a recognised measure of memory and mental function) had vastly improved.

The lowdown on phospholipids

Although your body can make phospholipids, getting some extra from your diet is even better. The richest sources of phospholipids in the average diet are egg yolks and organ meats. Nowadays we eat much less of both than we did a few decades ago. Since egg phobia set in, amid the unfounded fears that dietary cholesterol was the major cause of heart disease, our intake of phospholipids has gone down dramatically. And at the same time, the number of people suffering from memory and concentration problems has gone up.

Now you can understand why lions and other animals at the top of the food chain eat the organs and brain first. Foxes are one of the most adaptive of all animals in Britain. Their favourite meal is a chicken head. They're not stupid.

Go for gold – eat eggs

But we are stupid – or at least we are in danger of becoming so unless we include phospholipids in our diet. One way to do this is to eat more eggs. But aren't they high in fat and cholesterol? Although eggs do contain cholesterol, eating them doesn't raise your blood cholesterol level. In any event, cholesterol is essential for good health. Your brain contains vast amounts of it and it is used to make the sex hormones oestrogen, progesterone and testosterone.

The kind of fat in an egg depends on what you feed the chicken. As we learnt earlier, essential fats are good for you. If you feed it a diet rich in essential omega-3 fats, for example flax seeds or fishmeal, you get an egg high in omega-3. An egg is as healthy as the chicken that laid it. As long as you don't fry them, eggs are a great brain food, and the richest dietary source of choline.

A real wonder drug – lecithin

Lecithin is the best source of phospholipids, and is widely available in health food shops, sold either as lecithin granules or capsules. 'Lecithin is practically a wonder drug as far as cognitive impairment is concerned,' says Dr Dharma Singh Khalsa, author of *Brain Longevity* and an expert in nutrition and its role in enhancing memory.

The ideal daily intake to keep your brain in top shape is 5g of lecithin, or half this if you take 'high PC' (phosphatidyl choline) lecithin. The easiest and cheapest way to take this is to add a tablespoon of lecithin, or a heaped teaspoon of high-PC lecithin, to your cereal in the morning. Or you can take lecithin supplements. Most capsules provide 1200mg, so you would need four a day. In case you were wondering, lecithin doesn't make you fat. In fact, quite the opposite: it helps the body digest fat.

I'm going to explain all about the vital role phospholipids play in keeping your brain healthy in Chapter 10, but for now I want to make sure you are getting enough in your diet by:

- Adding a tablespoon of lecithin granules, or a heaped teaspoon of high-PC lecithin, to your cereal every day
- Or eating an egg – preferably free-range, organic and high in omega-3s (the omega-3 content of eggs is determined by the diet of the hen that laid it – check labelling for details. Organic hens are not necessarily fed on a high omega-3 diet)
- Or supplementing a brain food formula providing phosphatidyl choline and phosphatidyl serine.

Amino Acid Check

- [ ] Do you eat less than one portion of protein-rich foods (meat, dairy, fish, eggs, tofu) each day?
- [ ] Do you eat less than two servings of vegetable sources of protein (beans, lentils, quinoa, seeds, nuts, wholegrains) each day?
- [ ] If you're vegetarian, do you rarely combine different protein foods such as those mentioned above?
- [ ] Are you very physically active or do you work out a lot?
- [ ] Do you suffer from anxiety, depression or irritability?
- [ ] Are you frequently tired or lacking in motivation?
- [ ] Do you sometimes lose concentration or have poor memory?
- [ ] Do you have very low blood pressure?
- [ ] Do your hair and nails grow slowly?
- [ ] Are you constantly hungry or do you frequently get indigestion?

If you ticked five or more boxes, the chances are you're not getting enough protein, which provides amino acids.

Amino acids are themselves the building blocks of protein in the body, and they improve communication in the brain. As we've seen, the messages sent from one cell to another are called neurotransmitters, and you could say that the letters in the words they contain are built from amino acids.

A deficiency in amino acids isn't at all uncommon, and it can give rise to depression, apathy and lack of motivation, an inability to relax, poor memory and concentration. Supplementing amino acids has been proven to correct all these problems. For example, a form of the amino acid called tryptophan has proven more effective in double-blind trials than the best antidepressant drugs.[24] The amino acid tyrosine improves mental and physical performance under stress better than coffee.[25] And the amino acid GABA, which is itself a neurotransmitter, is involved in reducing anxiety.[26]

Protein power

Protein is vital. Since almost all neurotransmitters are made from it, you can influence how you feel by giving yourself an ideal quantity and quality of protein every day. By taking this in an easily absorbed form it can be put to good use by your body and brain. The better the quality and 'usability' of the protein you eat, the less you actually need to be optimally nourished.

The quality of a protein is determined by its balance of amino acids. Though there are 23 amino acids from which the body can build everything from a neurotransmitter to a neuron, you actually need to eat only the eight so-called 'essential' amino acids, because the body can make the rest from these. The better the balance of amino acids – expressed as a unit called an NPU, which stands for 'net protein usability' – the more you can make use of the protein.

The chart opposite shows the top 24 individual foods and food combinations in terms of NPUs, or protein quality. Combining beans with rice, for example, is a great way of increasing protein content. It also shows how much of a food, or food combination, you need to eat to get 20g of protein. A man needs to eat the equivalent of 3 to 4 of these servings, while a woman needs to eat 2 to 3, every day.

A typical day's allotment of protein for a man might therefore include an egg for breakfast (10g), a 200g/7oz salmon steak for lunch (40g), and a serving of beans with dinner (20g).

For a vegetarian, a typical day's worth might be a small tub of yoghurt and a heaped tablespoon of seeds on an oat-based cereal for breakfast (20g), and a 275g/10oz serving of tofu (20g) and vegetable steam-fry, served with either a cup of the protein-rich grain quinoa (20g), or a serving of beans with rice (20g) as part of dinner. The trick for vegetarians is to eat 'seed' foods – that is, foods that would grow if you planted them. These include seeds, nuts, beans, lentils, peas, maize or the germ of grains such as wheat or oat. 'Flower' foods such as broccoli or cauliflower are also relatively rich in protein.

Note that the cup measures indicated are imperial, not American.

Packed with Protein: the Top 24

Food	Percentage of calories as protein	How much for 20g (¾oz)	Protein quality (NPU)
Grains/Pulses			
Quinoa	16	100g (3½oz)/1 cup dry weight	Excellent
Tofu	40	275g (10oz)/1 packet	Reasonable
Maize	4	500g (1lb 2oz)/4 cups cooked weight	Reasonable
Brown rice	5	400g (14oz)/3 cups cooked weight	Excellent
Chickpeas	22	115g (4oz)/⅔ cup cooked weight	Reasonable
Lentils	28	85g (3oz)/1 cup cooked weight	Reasonable
Fish/meat			
Tuna, canned	61	85g (3oz)/1 small tin	Excellent
Cod	60	35g (1¼oz)/1 very small piece	Excellent
Salmon	50	100g (3½oz)/1 small piece	Excellent
Sardines	49	100g (3½oz)/1 baked	Excellent
Chicken	63	75g (2½oz)/1 small roasted breast	Excellent

Food	Percentage of calories as protein	How much for 20g (¾oz)	Protein quality (NPU)
Nuts/seeds			
Sunflower seeds	15	185g (6½oz)/1 cup	Reasonable
Pumpkin seeds	21	75g (2½oz)/½ cup	Reasonable
Cashew nuts	12	115g (4oz)/1 cup	Reasonable
Almonds	13	115g (4oz)/1 cup	Reasonable
Eggs/dairy foods			
Eggs	34	115g (4oz)/2 medium	Excellent
Yoghurt, natural	22	450g (1lb)/3 small pots	Excellent
Cottage cheese	49	125g (4½oz)/1 small pot	Excellent
Vegetables			
Peas, frozen	26	250g (9oz)/2 cups	Reasonable
Other beans	20	200g (7oz)/2 cups	Reasonable
Broccoli	50	40g (1½oz)/½ cup	Reasonable
Spinach	49	40g (1½oz)/⅔ cup	Reasonable
Combinations			
Lentils and rice	18	125g (4½oz)/small cup dry weight	Excellent
Beans and rice	15	125g (4½oz)/small cup dry weight	Excellent

If after reading this chart, you were astonished at the amount of maize or brown rice you'd have to eat to get 20g of protein, please don't imagine I'm suggesting you eat mounds of them to top up your daily protein requirements. It's best to focus on the higher protein foods for your daily needs, and continue to eat sensible portions of foods with low to moderate protein content. It's just good to know that some 'seed' carbohydrate foods such as maize and brown rice have protein content, as this does help you keep your diet protein-rich.

Supplementing amino acids

While eating protein is the best way to start to get essential amino acids into your diet, supplementing amino acids is the best way to correct neurotransmitter imbalances. I'll explain how to do this in Part 2, but for now, here are some general guidelines to help ensure you have an optimal intake of amino acids – the alphabet of mind and mood.

- Have three servings of the protein-rich foods shown opposite a day, if you are a man, and two if you are a woman.
- Choose good vegetable protein sources, including beans, lentils, quinoa, tofu, 'seed' vegetables such as maize, and 'flower' vegetables such as broccoli and cauliflower.
- If eating animal protein, choose lean meat or preferably fish, organic whenever possible.

Intelligent Nutrient Check

- [ ] Do you eat fewer than five servings of fresh fruits and vegetables (excluding potato) every day?
- [ ] Do you eat less than one portion of dark green vegetables a day?
- [ ] Do you eat fewer than three portions of fresh or dried tropical fruit a week?
- [ ] Do you eat seeds (pumpkin, sunflower, sesame) or unroasted nuts less than three times a week?
- [ ] Are you currently not taking a multivitamin/mineral supplement every day?

cont. overleaf

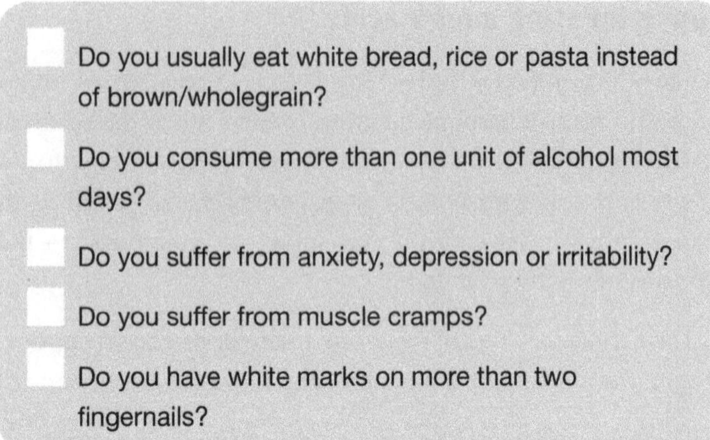

- [ ] Do you usually eat white bread, rice or pasta instead of brown/wholegrain?
- [ ] Do you consume more than one unit of alcohol most days?
- [ ] Do you suffer from anxiety, depression or irritability?
- [ ] Do you suffer from muscle cramps?
- [ ] Do you have white marks on more than two fingernails?

If you ticked five or more boxes, the chances are you're not getting enough of vital vitamins and minerals for your brain.

In every great production, there are hundreds of people 'behind the scenes' supporting the main player. With your brain, it's vitamins and minerals. One of their central roles is to help turn glucose into energy, amino acids into neurotransmitters, simple essential fats into more complex fats like GLA or DHA and prostaglandins, and choline and serine into phospholipids. They help build and rebuild the brain and nervous system and keep everything running smoothly. They are some of your brain's best friends.

So the sooner you start optimally nourishing your brain, the better. Every one of the 50 known essential nutrients, with the exception of vitamin D, plays a major role in promoting mental health. Here are some of the key ones, including symptoms you might experience if you're deficient, and the best foods to eat to help you get enough.

The Key Nutrients for Intelligence

Nutrient	Effects of deficiency	Food sources
B1	Poor concentration and attention	Wholegrains, vegetables
B3	Depression, psychosis	Wholegrains, vegetables
B5	Poor memory, stress	Wholegrains, vegetables
B6	Irritability, poor memory, depression, stress	Wholegrains, bananas
Folic acid	Anxiety, depression, psychosis	Green leafy vegetables
B12	Confusion, poor memory, psychosis	Meat, fish, dairy products, eggs
Vitamin C	Depression, psychosis	Vegetables and fresh fruit
Magnesium	Irritability, insomnia, depression	Green vegetables, nuts, seeds
Manganese	Dizziness, convulsions	Nuts, seeds, tropical fruit, tea
Zinc	Confusion, blank mind, depression, loss of appetite, lack of motivation and concentration	Oysters, nuts, seeds, fish

The Bs and C

The B group of vitamins is vital for mental health. A deficiency in any one of the eight B vitamins will rapidly affect how you think and feel. This is because they are water-soluble and rapidly pass through the body, and out of it – so we need a regular intake throughout the day. Also, since the brain uses a very large amount of these nutrients, a short-term deficiency will affect mental abilities. While the deficiency symptoms of B vitamins are well known, we still do not know exactly why many of the symptoms occur. Each B vitamin has so many functions in the brain and nervous system there are many logical explanations, but few hard proofs. Many people choose to safeguard against deficiency by taking a B complex supplement or a multivitamin every day.

Vitamin C is another star in this context – it does much more than stop you from getting a cold! It has many roles to play in the brain, including helping to balance neurotransmitters. I'll be explaining why these are so important for your brain in Chapters 7 and 8.

Minerals – Nature's tranquillisers

Popping a mineral may be the last thing you'd think of doing when you're feeling anxious, edgy and unable to relax. Yet calcium and magnesium will do the trick, by helping to relax nerve and muscle cells. A lack of either of these minerals can also make you more nervous, irritable and aggressive. Most of all, they help you to sleep.

Your brain also needs manganese, a mineral found mainly in seeds, nuts and grains and tropical fruit such as bananas and pineapples. But the most important mineral of all, and the one we're most commonly deficient in, is zinc. It's well worth supplementing extra.

I'll explain why these minerals are so important for protecting against Alzheimer's in Chapter 8, but for now, here are some guidelines to help ensure you have an optimal intake of vitamins and minerals to keep your brain in top shape:

- Eat at least five, and ideally seven, servings of fresh fruit and vegetables a day.

- Eat nuts and seeds regularly, and choose wholefoods, such as wholegrains, lentils, beans and brown rice, rather than refined food.
- Supplement a multivitamin and mineral that gives you at least 25mg of all the B vitamins, 10mcg of B12, 200mcg of folic acid, 200mg of magnesium, 3mg of manganese and 10mg of zinc.

You'll now have a good idea about the areas of your diet or lifestyle that are taxing your brain, and are almost ready to look at the 10 proven ways of helping to minimise your chances of developing age-related memory decline and Alzheimer's. But, before doing so there's one more step, and that is to make sure both of your brains are well nourished.

That's right – you have two brains.

The gut–brain connection

It used to be thought that all our thinking was done by neurons in the brain. We now know that the digestive system contains 100 million neurons, and produces as many neurotransmitters as the brain does. The gut produces two-thirds of the body's serotonin, the 'happy' neurotransmitter, for instance.

So in essence, when you eat, you're feeding two brains. Every time you eat something it sends signals to the brain because the gut and the brain are in permanent communication. This is why the right foods can make you happy and the wrong foods can make you feel anxious or depressed.

As one Harvard Medical School gastroenterologist once said, 'Having a good stomach and set of bowels is as important to human happiness as a large amount of brains.' Good nutrition isn't just about what you eat, it's also about what you can digest and absorb.

The older you are, the worse your ability to absorb certain nutrients becomes. Vitamin B12 becomes harder to absorb as you get older – one reason why older people need much more than the RDA (a measly 1mcg) to stay healthy. I'd recommend everyone, at any age, to supplement 10mcg a day as a matter of course. One recent study found that supplements of 50mcg were effective in restoring normal B12 status in people over the age of 50, whereas supplements of 10mcg were no more effective than a placebo.[27]

One reason for this problem with absorption is a lack of sufficient stomach acid. Getting B12 into your system depends on something called 'intrinsic factor', produced in the stomach. To break protein down properly, and make use of the amino acids that you need to keep your neurotransmitter balance at peak, you also need stomach acid. Stomach acid production, in turn, depends on zinc, while protein digestion depends on zinc and vitamin B6. Making sure you have enough of all these nutrients not only gives you more, but helps you absorb more, from your diet.

Now you're ready to read about the 10 most important steps you need to take to protect you from ever developing dementia or Alzheimer's. If you follow them what you'll find is that there's immediate gratification too – a vast, and fast, improvement in mind, mood and memory.

PART 2

Ten Ways to Enhance Your Memory

Ten simple steps are all it takes to protect your brain and enhance your memory and concentration. Each is based on solid science, and represents a piece of the jigsaw that shows why some people develop Alzheimer's disease, and some don't. Making these steps part of your daily routine is your best bet for staying free of age-related cognitive decline.

7

The Homocysteine Connection

THE SINGLE MOST exciting discovery in Alzheimer's prevention is that the amino acid homocysteine is involved in the development of the disease. Knowing your level is one of the best ways to determine your risk before symptoms develop. But more importantly, this is a highly reversible risk factor, involving no recourse to expensive drugs or procedures – just simple dietary changes and B vitamin supplementation. We'll see how to put it all together in this chapter.

You'd think that such an important discovery would be welcomed with open arms by the medical community and governments alike. The sad truth is that, with no patentable or profitable treatment involved in lowering homocysteine levels, scientists are finding it hard to get their studies funded. And once funded, it isn't always easy for them to publish their findings in mainstream journals, since they are dominated by editors who believe the current dogmas.

On top of all this, many pharmaceutical companies are funding very poorly designed trials using B vitamins, some using only folic acid, others doses that are too low. It's almost as if they would like to slow down the progress of this breakthrough. And it is true that the discovery of the homocysteine link will ultimately be bad news for the pharmaceutical industry's profits from competitive drugs such as the acetylcholinesterase inhibitor Aricept. Such drugs generate billions of pounds in profits, and you can be sure the companies making them will protect their turf.

All this means that you are more likely to find out about this vitally important discovery from reading a book like this than from your doctor. In some countries such as Germany, where they run millions of tests a year, homocysteine is routinely measured. In the UK, few GPs are testing it. In fact, despite over 14,000 studies now published in scientific and medical journals, chances are you've never even heard of homocysteine. I'd like to tell you the whole story so you can judge for yourself.

Let's start at the beginning.

Homocysteine – what it is and what it does

In Part 1 we discovered that homocysteine is a type of amino acid produced by the body and found in the blood that, ideally, should be present in very low quantities. Problems arise, however, if you are not optimally nourished: homocysteine can accumulate in the blood, increasing the risk for over 50 diseases including heart attacks, strokes, certain cancers, osteoporosis, depression and Alzheimer's disease.

One in two people in Britain have high homocysteine levels. But the good news is that this new and important risk factor can be reversed in weeks.

Homocysteine is produced from another amino acid, methionine, which is found in normal dietary protein. In its turn, homocysteine itself is normally turned by your body into one of two beneficial substances. These are glutathione (the body's most important antioxidant), and SAMe, which as we've seen is a very important type of 'intelligent' nutrient for both brain and body.

Problems arise when you don't have optimal amounts of B vitamins in your diet. Then, the enzymes that turn homocysteine into these beneficial substances don't work well enough. Your homocysteine can't be converted, so your levels of it rise dangerously. (See figure opposite.)

To make matters more complex, it has been discovered that approximately 1 in 10 people have an inherited genetic mutation that makes them more prone to higher homocysteine levels than other people. This means that one of the cortical methylation enzymes, known as MTHFR, doesn't work so well. Luckily, studies show that larger daily intakes of B12 and folic acid can help to make the deficient enzyme work better.

While the importance of antioxidants is now well established, the new buzzword in Alzheimer's prevention is methylation – the body process we encountered on page 14. The body's ability to maintain chemical balance hinges upon its ability to add or subtract molecules called methyl groups. This is how we turn one body chemical into another. To make this real, let's say that you're riding your bike down a narrow road and a car pulls out right in front of you. You have to make a quick decision to save your life, and your body responds by adding a methyl group to noradrenalin to produce adrenalin – which kickstarts you into swift action. This kind of chemical reaction occurs a billion times every couple of seconds, keeping all your body chemistry in balance. If your homocysteine level is low then you are good at doing this.

If there was one measure of your antioxidant 'IQ', it would be the level of glutathione inside your cells (we'll discuss this in detail in the next chapter). All those antoxidants you eat and supplement every day have the greatest effect if they ultimately raise intracellular glutathione. If your homocysteine level is low then

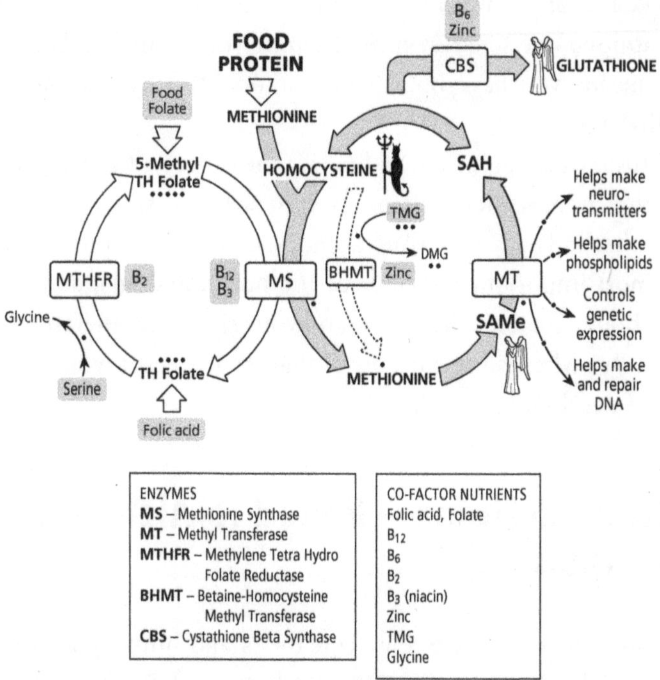

Figure 11. The homocysteine pathway: we all make homocysteine from eating protein. Normally, it is quickly turned into SAMe or glutathione, two essential and health-promoting substances in the body. But, if you lack enough of the nutrients such as B2, B6, B12, folic acid, zinc or TMG, the enzymes (shown in white boxes) that convert homocysteine into SAMe or glutathione don't work well enough and you end up accumulating toxic homocysteine. See www.patrickholford.com/methylationcycle for an animated version of this diagram

you'll have a healthy amount of glutathione protecting your body and brain.

Similarly, if there was one measure of your methyl 'IQ' it would be the level of SAMe inside your cells. This is because SAMe can easily donate a methyl group, or accept one back, keeping the body's biochemistry flexible. Normally, both SAMe and glutathione are made from the amino acid methionine in our diet, via homocysteine. However, if the conversion of homocysteine is blocked in any way, homocysteine levels go up and SAMe and glutathione levels go down. So, keeping your homocysteine level low means you have both a high antioxidant 'IQ' and a high methyl 'IQ'.

This is only half of the bad news. The other half is the discovery that homocysteine damages your arteries, your brain, and DNA itself. That's why your homocysteine level is theoretically the most important indicator of the health and adaptability of your body's total biochemistry, and your risk of degenerative diseases. But where's the hard proof that it's the best predictor of a risk of developing Alzheimer's?

Homocysteine – linked to Alzheimer's in 1998

The first firm link between Alzheimer's and homocysteine was reported in 1998, by Dr Robert Clarke and Professor David Smith from the University of Oxford, and Professor Helga Refsum, now at the University of Oslo, as part of OPTIMA (Oxford Project to Investigate Memory and Ageing). The researchers discovered high levels of homocysteine in the blood of patients who, after death, were proven to have Alzheimer's via examination of the brain.[28]

Since then, many different research groups have found high homocysteine levels in people suffering both age-related mental decline and Alzheimer's. For example, a research group in Italy found that having a raised homocysteine level (above 15 μmol/l) doubled an older person's chances of developing dementia and Alzheimer's over a four year period.[29] A research group in the US reported the same findings in 2005 – the higher the homocysteine the greater was the risk of cognitive decline in older men.[30]

To date, 70 out of 77 studies involving over 35,000 people have found a clear association between increasing homocysteine levels predicting increased risk of cognitive impairment and dementia or Alzheimer's.[31]

More recently, a growing number of indicators of Alzheimer's-related degeneration in the brain have been shown to be directly linked to homocysteine levels.[32] For instance, as Alzheimer's progresses the width of the hippocampus, a vital part of the brain associated with learning and memory, shrinks. The width of the hippocampus is directly related to homocysteine levels.[33]

At this point you might start to switch off, thinking, 'I don't have Alzheimer's so this isn't relevant to me.' But what has been discovered is that both the changes in the brain and rising homocysteine levels happen decades before the development of any noticeable Alzheimer's symptoms. So keeping tabs on your homocysteine levels allows you to pre-diagnose the risk for Alzheimer's, and do something simple to reverse it now, before you develop more serious symptoms.

While these discoveries may provide an important clue to the prevention of Alzheimer's, they don't prove that high homocysteine actually causes Alzheimer's. High homocysteine can cause cardiovascular disease, poor blood circulation to the brain and silent strokes (which happens when smaller blood vessels in the brain become blocked); and it can indicate low levels of B vitamins, poor methylation and depleted glutathione. All these conditions are linked to an increased risk of Alzheimer's. But how do you know that homocysteine actually causes Alzheimer's, rather than just predicting it?[34] Some researchers have argued that the high homocysteine score found in Alzheimer's sufferers is simply showing the person has one of these related conditions, such as cardiovascular disease or a folic acid deficiency, rather than proving a direct link.

A recent study from the School of Medicine at the University of California, Davis, is a case in point. Researchers compared 43 patients with Alzheimer's to 37 without. They found a stronger association between a high homocysteine score and cardiovascular disease, in both groups, than between a high homocysteine score and Alzheimer's. They also found that those with low levels of B6 in the blood were more likely to have high homocysteine levels.[35] The researchers concluded that high levels of homocysteine in the blood of Alzheimer's patients appeared to relate to vascular disease, not Alzheimer's. In addition, they reported that 'low vitamin B6 status is prevalent in patients with Alzheimer's. It remains to be determined if elevated homocysteine and/or low vitamin B6 status directly influences Alzheimer's pathogenesis or progression.'

This is one of those 'chicken or egg' situations that some researchers are beginning to fully unravel, however. The evidence to date strongly favours the position that homocysteine, independent of vascular disease, is a major risk factor for Alzheimer's. Of course, if you have both high homocysteine and vascular disease, you are even worse off.[36]

Does high homocysteine cause Alzheimer's?

So the big question is which comes first – a high homocysteine level or Alzheimer's? Doctors from the Boston University School of Medicine neurology department wanted to answer it by determining whether homocysteine actually precedes mental decline, or occurs as a result of dementia-related B vitamin deficiencies.

Their study looked at 1,092 people who had an average age of 76, did not have dementia and had already taken part in another study measuring their homocysteine levels, eight years earlier. The researchers again measured their homocysteine, and then kept track of their mental health over the next eight years.

During that time, 111 developed dementia, 83 of whom were diagnosed with Alzheimer's. The findings revealed that the higher the homocysteine levels preceding any symptoms of mental decline, the greater the risk of later developing dementia. In those with a homocysteine score of more than 14 units, the risk of Alzheimer's almost doubled.[37] They concluded that 'an increased homocysteine level is a strong, independent risk factor for the development of dementia and Alzheimer's disease'. This powerfully suggests that optimum nutrition could, at the very least, halve your risk of developing Alzheimer's in later years by lowering your homocysteine levels.

More recently, evidence has emerged that even before there is evidence of declining mental function in so-called 'healthy' elderly individuals, high homocysteine also predicts physical degeneration in certain parts of the brain.[38–9] These findings are being echoed by research around the world.[40]

In Scotland, researchers have found that a reduction in mental performance in old age is strongly associated with high homocysteine and low levels of vitamins B12 and folate. They studied people who had taken part in the Scottish Mental Surveys of 1932 and 1947, which surveyed childhood intelligence. And they found that while homocysteine was higher and mental performance weaker in the older group, the most mentally agile of either group had the highest levels of B vitamins and lowest levels of homocysteine. In the older group, high homocysteine accounted for a 7 to 8 per cent decline in mental performance.[41]

Homocysteine doesn't cause just mental deterioration. It also predicts physical deterioration. Research at the University of California, Los Angeles, has found that physical performance in older people, using tests of body strength, coordination, manual dexterity and gait, also declines as homocysteine levels increase.[42]

Whichever way you cut it, the accumulating evidence is pointing to a consistent pattern. The higher your homocysteine score and the lower your B vitamin status, the greater your chances of declining memory, poor concentration and judgement, lowered mood, physical degeneration and poor circulation to the brain.

How homocysteine damages the brain

Exactly how high homocysteine – and the inevitable B vitamin and SAMe deficiencies that always accompany it – might contribute to the kind of brain damage seen in Alzheimer's has become a subject of heated debate in scientific circles around the world.

In Japan, Dr Toshifumi Matsui and colleagues at Tohoku University conducted brain scans on 153 elderly people and checked them against each individual's homocysteine level. The evidence was clear – the higher the homocysteine, the greater the damage to the brain.[43] They also confirmed that high homocysteine levels were strongly correlated with low folic acid levels.

There's also evidence that homocysteine and its derivatives can activate certain receptors on the surface of nerve cells that result in the cell's death.[44–5] Another possible explanation is that homocysteine damages the microscopic blood vessels supplying critical brain regions, reducing blood supply and again, resulting in nerve cell death.[46] A research group at the Baylor University Metabolic Disease Center in Dallas, Texas, led by Dr Teodoro Bottiglieri – one of the world's leading experts on the connection between folate and mental illness – proposes that low levels of folate (which can lead to raised homocysteine levels) directly cause brain damage that triggers dementia and Alzheimer's. Their research has found that a third of those with both dementia and high homocysteine scores (above 14 units) are deficient in folate.[47] Dr David Snowdon at the University of Kentucky has also confirmed from autopsies that the lower the levels of serum folic acid, the greater the brain damage a person suffered.[48]

Alzheimer's sufferers also have less SAMe in their brains, as well as higher levels of homocysteine in their blood. SAMe, which as we've seen is derived from the methylation of homocysteine, is the brain's single most important methyl donor. As such it helps to produce and activate all sorts of neurotransmitters, including the memory enhancer acetylcholine – declining levels of which are another hallmark of Alzheimer's and a likely reason for declining memory.[49]

Recently, research has identified something you don't want too much of, called P-tau. This leads to the build up of neurofibrillary tangles, effectively nerve damage, which is one of the hallmarks of Alzheimer's. Once again, homocysteine is involved because having high homocysteine leads to the build up of toxic P-tau.[50] This might be one of the mechanisms by which homocysteine actually damages the brain, and why it is possible to prevent brain damage by lowering your homocysteine level.

Is Alzheimer's and memory decline arrestable?

But can you reverse the process of decay? This is the 64 million dollar question.

To answer it, I'd like to start by telling you about the work of a GP in Wales, Dr Andrew McCaddon. He started researching homocysteine more than a decade ago and has pioneered research in Alzheimer's treatment.

How B vitamins can stabilise Alzheimer's

It all began in 1990, when Dr Andrew McCaddon met a 59–year-old patient with a nine-year history of mental problems due to early-onset familial Alzheimer's disease. His patient had low B12 levels in the blood, but normal B12 absorption. Dr McCaddon noticed that other affected family members also had low vitamin B12 levels in their medical records.[51]

In 1992, he published a hypothesis describing how this deficiency might contribute to Alzheimer's, but he needed to test his theory.[52] Since B12 and folic acid are necessary for converting homocysteine to methionine, he predicted that

cont. overleaf

these patients with low levels of B12 or folic acid would have elevated blood levels of homocysteine. That is exactly what he found.[53] He also found that a person's homocysteine level was the best predictor of a decline in cognitive function.[54]

Since this early research he has gone on to prove that homocysteine levels increase as cognitive function declines – a finding now consistently being reported by other research groups.[55] He then started giving patients large amounts of B vitamins. This is what happened.

> In the beginning, we gave B12 and folic acid to patients with high homocysteine levels, but we didn't really get much improvement. We realized that in Alzheimer's and in vascular dementia, there's a lot of oxidative stress, which also impacts on homocysteine and methylation. So we started to give N-acetyl cysteine as well, which the brain uses to make glutathione, its primary anti-oxidant. That's when I started to see a difference.
>
> To date, I have six cases of people diagnosed with Alzheimer's who have not got worse. Often they report an improvement in general well-being and other aspects of mental health. For example, one lady has a clear improvement in her drawing ability.
>
> Another example is Mrs R. She developed cognitive impairment 10 years ago. Her husband became seriously concerned five years ago after she had gone shopping and couldn't find her way back home. He helplessly watched her get worse. When she came to see me, I tested her homocysteine level, which was very high, and gave her B12, folic acid and N-acetyl cysteine.
>
> Within six months she became calmer and started sleeping properly. When she went out, she knew where she was going. Her underlying personality is now back.

> She's friendly, she can cope, and her behaviour is good. In the words of her husband, 'We can sit, eat tea and biscuits, watch TV, and talk. I've got my wife back.' Her short-term memory isn't great, but she hasn't got any worse. This is exactly what we're seeing consistently – a halting of the course of the disease. People don't get worse.

Dr McCaddon's research has not only shown that the right amount and form of vitamins can arrest the progress of Alzheimer's in the small number of people treated so far. It has also shown that people with Alzheimer's may not use B12 properly, despite showing apparently normal levels in the blood.[56–7] One way round this B12 blockage is to give a special form of B12, either methylcobalamin or glutathionylcobalamine.[58]

Even though McCaddon's cases are encouraging they are still not definitive proof that giving homocysteine-lowering B vitamins can slow or reverse age-related memory decline and prevent you developing Alzheimer's and, if a person has it, stop it getting worse.

Two recent studies have been published on this subject. The first looked at the effects of giving homocysteine-lowering B vitamins to those already diagnosed as suffering from mild to moderate Alzheimer's.[59] The researchers gave 202 Alzheimer's patients B vitamins (daily 5mg of folic acid, 1,000μg of B12, and 25mg of B6) over a period of 18 months but found no overall difference compared with the 138 in the placebo group. However, when they divided the patients into those with high and low cognitive test scores at the start, those who had milder Alzheimer's did significantly respond; those taking the B vitamins hardly got worse over 15 months, while those on the placebo showed a steady decline. The average drop in homocysteine over the 18 months was from 9.1 to 6.8μmol/l. This study suggests that homocysteine-lowering B vitamins can, at least, slow down Alzheimer's substantially in the early stages, but that when the disease has reached the moderately severe stage it may be too late.

Perhaps even more important is whether homocysteine-lowering B vitamins can prevent Alzheimer's from ever developing. A study headed by Professor David Smith from the University of Oxford studied the effects of giving homocysteine-lowering B vitamins (folic acid 800mcg, B6 20mg, and B12 500mcg) to 270 people with age-related memory decline. They also tested their homocysteine levels and did an MRI brain scan in most of the participants at the beginning and end of the 24–month placebo controlled trial. The results showed that in the placebo group the higher the homocysteine level the greater was the rate of brain shrinkage, with those above 13μmol/l (in the top quarter of the population) having a rate of shrinkage of 1.5 per cent per year compared to 0.8 per cent in those with a homocysteine level of below 9.5μmol/l (in the bottom quarter of the population). The effect of giving the B vitamins on brain shrinkage was remarkable, especially among those with raised homocysteine levels: in those with levels above 13μmol/l the B vitamins led to a 53 per cent reduction in the rate of shrinkage. Also, when they looked specifically at which areas of the brain had reduced shrinkage, they found that those with raised homocysteine levels at the start of the trial, who were on the placebos, had over eight times more shrinkage in the medial temporal lobe (the area that diagnoses Alzheimer's) than those on the B vitamins. Also, those on the B vitamins had virtually no further decline in memory.[60]

Previous work by this group had shown that brain shrinkage is associated with a person's B12 status; those with low-B12 status showing more rapid shrinkage, which is one of the early signs of Alzheimer's.

B12 and folic acid – are you really getting enough?

B12 deficiency is common among people over the age of 60 but it appears that even levels in the low–normal range may be harmful. In a study of 61 to 87 year olds, the lower the level the greater was the brain size shrinkage.[61] None of these subjects was B12 deficient.

However, low B12 status is rarely properly checked for and there are good grounds for making it a routine test, along with homocysteine, for anyone over the age of 60. This is because its ability to be absorbed becomes worse with age. The usual means of checking is to measure one's plasma B12 levels, but this is a very crude measure and it is becoming clear that having a level in the low end of the so-called 'normal' range is associated with worsening memory. In fact, in Japan they treat a level below 500ng/l; in the UK, the cut off point is often 150ng/l. Much more accurate is a test called MMA (methylmalonic acid), which is a more reliable marker for B12 deficiency and becomes high if you are deficient. Another alternative is to test HoloTransCobalamin(HoloTC) which, if low, indicates deficiency. An MMA test is more widely available. This chemical only accumulates if you are deficient in B12, or not using it efficiently. The greater the B12 deficiency, according to these tests, the worse is a person's memory scores, the higher is their homocysteine level and the greater is their risk for dementia or Alzheimer's.[62–3]

If you want to be sure of your B12 status it is best to get your MMA level tested. This should be below 0.37μmol/l. If your homocysteine level is also high it is wise to assume you are not getting enough vitamin B12.

B12 is only found in animal foods, such as meat, fish, eggs and milk. But only increasing the intake of fish and milk is linked to increasing B12 levels.[64] Increasing meat and eggs does not seem to be anything like as effective for improving your B12 status. My advice is to eat more fish (in Chapter 10 the reasons for this will become most obvious) and also to supplement at least 10mcg at any age, 50mcg if you are over 50, and 500mcg or more (see page 97) if you have a raised homocysteine level.

The reason for recommending this seemingly very high level,

given that the RDA is only 2.5µg, is that only these kind of daily intakes help to correct deficiency. That's what a group of researchers in Holland found when they investigated how much B12 you need to take in to correct mild B12 deficiency. Only doses of 647 to 1032µg of B12 were associated with correcting deficiency. In their words, 'the lowest dose of oral B12 required to normalize mild B12 deficiency is more than 200 times greater than the RDA [2.5µg]'.[65] So much for a 'well balanced diet' giving you all the nutrients you need!

The other homocysteine-lowering B vitamin you really need to make sure you are getting enough of is folic acid, which works with B12 to raise your methyl IQ. The higher your intake, the lower your risk. One recent study found that, among older people, those in the top quarter of folic acid intake had half the risk of Alzheimer's.[66]

A study conducted by Jane Durga at Wageningen University in Holland, gave 818 people aged 50 to 75 either a dummy pill or a vitamin containing 800mcg of folic acid a day. That's almost three times the RDA and the equivalent of 2½ pounds of strawberries a day – more than you can reasonably eat. Three years later, different aspects of intelligence were measured. On memory tests, the supplement users had scores comparable to people 5.5 years younger. On tests of cognitive speed, they performed as well as people 1.9 years younger.[67]

As vital as folic acid is for good methylation it is still only one of six methylation nutrients (the others being B2, B6, B12, zinc and TMG) that should always be taken together. There are good reasons for this. For example, the classic sign of either folic acid or B12 deficiency is tiredness. If a person is low in B12, but supplements folic acid, often the tiredness goes away but the more insidious nerve damage caused by a lack of B12, continues under the surface.

In fact, a recent study in the US found that elderly people with low B12 intakes (poor diet) but high folic acid (from fortification) were five times more likely to have memory decline.[68] This is probably because extra folic acid can hide the blood symptoms of low B12.

I never give folic acid alone to anyone, not even to a pregnant woman. The best way to discover how much you need is to test your homocysteine level. Otherwise I'd recommend supplementing folic acid as part of a multivitamin containing at least 10mcg of B12, 25mg of B6 and 10mg of zinc.

Homocysteine – the story so far

In summary, what we already know is that:

- People with Alzheimer's consistently have high homocysteine, and low B12 and folate levels.[69–70]
- High homocysteine, as well as low folate and B12 status, predict a risk of developing Alzheimer's and age-related memory problems.
- High homocysteine is associated with more rapid progression of the disease and more rapid shrinkage of the brain.[71]
- Homocysteine levels correlate with a degree of brain damage – and the kind of damage that suggests the development of dementia and Alzheimer's.
- High homocysteine can damage both the brain and arteries, leading to poor blood supply to the brain.
- Giving B vitamins that lower homocysteine both arrests abnormal brain shrinkage in those with age-related memory and arrests memory decline in those with mild, or early stage Alzheimer's.
- Case studies also show that giving increased amounts of homocysteine-lowering nutrients seems to arrest the progression of Alzheimer's. (For an example see the case study overleaf.)

Case study

Mary, at 75, complained to her GP that she had been feeling generally unwell, tearful, breathless and had the occasional sensation of a lump in her throat. The doctor ran some tests but didn't find anything 'wrong' with her and concluded that her symptoms were anxiety related. Three years later, she visited her GP again, complaining that for several months she had been feeling tired, lethargic and shaky, that her sleeping patterns and mood weren't very good and that she still felt generally unwell. Her only obvious physical symptoms were cracks at the corners of her mouth. Further blood tests were run which found extremely low levels of vitamin B12. She began having monthly injections of this vitamin and she felt much better, her mood lifted and the condition of her mouth improved.

However, within four years she started to develop problems with her short-term memory, especially when it came to remembering names and putting names to faces. She also became tearful again. Mental tests concluded that she had early signs of dementia, with associated depression. She was prescribed antidepressants and offered social support. Over the following six months her depression lifted, but her memory problems continued to get worse. A year later, a repeat mental test confirmed that her mental faculties were in decline.

At this point a daily dose of a nutrient called N-acetyl cysteine (NAC) was prescribed, in addition to her continued regular vitamin B12 injections. Glutathione can be made in the body from NAC, and glutathione helps the body use vitamin B12 more effectively. Within two weeks, her husband had seen a definite improvement in her memory, including being able to put names to faces. She also felt generally better. Repeat mental tests confirmed these improvements.

Get a handle on your homocysteine – now

Measure your level

The implication of all this research is that it's a very good idea to start by measuring your homocysteine level now. This is easy to do at home, with a test kit (see Resources, page 249).

Homocysteine is measured in micromol/l, written as µmol/l. We used to think a 'high' level was above 15 units (µmol/l). This is what increases your risk of a heart attack and doubles your Alzheimer's risk. Now, however, levels as low as 7 units are being linked to increased disease risk. Basically, there's no official safe level and no guarantee that the diet and supplements you are currently taking are keeping homocysteine at bay.

Up to 30 per cent of people with a history of heart disease have a homocysteine level above 14 units. The average level in Britain is 10.5. However, experts believe that a level below 7 units is ideal. If you have any of the associated risk factors listed in the two checklists overleaf, it's especially important to get tested. Since homocysteine does go up with age, if you are pursuing optimal health and minimal risk of developing any disease, including Alzheimer's, my rule of thumb is to keep your 'H' score below your age, divided by ten. So, if you are 80, keep your level below 8.

The H signs and symptoms – check yourself out

If you have five or more of the symptoms listed overleaf, it's almost a certainty that your homocysteine is moderately to very high (9 to 15, if not higher).

- [ ] Are you tired a lot of the time?
- [ ] Is your stamina, or ability to keep going, noticeably decreasing?
- [ ] Are you having a hard time keeping your weight stable?
- [ ] Do you often experience physical pain, be it arthritis, muscle aches or migraines?
- [ ] Do you get frequent colds?
- [ ] Is your eyesight deteriorating?
- [ ] Is your mental clarity or concentration decreasing?
- [ ] Are you experiencing more sleeping problems?
- [ ] Is your memory on the decline?
- [ ] Are you often depressed?
- [ ] Do you average two or more alcoholic beverages daily?
- [ ] Do you drink more than three cups of coffee daily?
- [ ] Do you smoke cigarettes?
- [ ] Are you a strict vegetarian?
- [ ] Do you eat red meat at least once a day?

Has your first-degree family (mother, father, brothers and sisters) suffered from any of the following?

- [ ] Heart disease, especially before 50 years of age
- [ ] Strokes
- [ ] Alzheimer's disease
- [ ] Abnormal blood clots

- [ ] Osteoporosis
- [ ] Cancer
- [ ] Severe depression (especially in women)
- [ ] Elevated homocysteine levels

Supplement the right nutrients

The most powerful and quickest way to restore a normal H score, below 7 units, is to supplement specific homocysteine-lowering nutrients. These include vitamins B2, B6, B12, folic acid, trimethylglycine (TMG) and zinc.

Here are the guidelines. If your H score is below 7, you can achieve these kinds of levels from a high-strength multivitamin. However, if your score is above 7 you will need to also take a specific supplement containing all these nutrients, designed to normalise your homocysteine level. Do re-check your homocysteine level and adjust your supplements accordingly. Higher doses of folic acid are not advisable unless your homocysteine level is high since there is some evidence that high folic acid intakes can speed up colo-rectal cancer progression. If you have active cancer it is best to take no more than 200mcg.

Nutrient	No risk	Very low risk	At risk	High risk	Very high risk
	Below 7	7–9.4	9.5–11.4	11.5–14.9	Above 15
Folic acid	200mcg	200mcg	400mcg	800mcg	800mcg
Methyl-B12	10mcg	250mcg	500mcg	500mcg	1000mcg
B6	10mg	20mg	25mg	25mg	50mg
B2	5mg	10mg	15mg	20mg	25mg
TMG		500mg	750mg	1000mg	2000mg
Zinc	5mg	5mg	10mg	15mg	20mg
NAC/ Glutathione		50mg	250mg	500mg	750mg

The current vogue in medicine is to recommend taking folic acid alone. Described in the *British Medical Journal* as 'the leading contender for panacea of the 21st century', folic acid alone is far less effective than the right nutrients in combination. The amount you need also depends on your current homocysteine level. One study found homocysteine scores were reduced by 17 per cent on high-dose folic acid alone, 19 per cent on vitamin B12 alone, 57 per cent on folic acid plus B12, and 60 per cent on folic acid, B12 and B6.[72] All this was achieved in three weeks!

However, even better results would have been achieved by including TMG. This is the best methyl donor to supplement, better even than SAMe. This is because only it can immediately donate a methyl group to homocysteine, thus detoxifying it. In one New Zealand study, the homocysteine scores of patients with chronic kidney failure and very high homocysteine levels were reduced by a further 18 per cent when 4g of TMG was given, along with 50mg of vitamin B6 and 5000mcg of folate, compared to patients taking just B6 and folate.[73] At the Brain Bio Centre we achieve, on average, reductions in high homocysteine scores of over 50 per cent in eight to twelve weeks with the combination of these nutrients, plus diet!

Some companies produce combinations of these nutrients (see Resources, page 251). These are the most cost-effective supplements for restoring a healthy homocysteine level.

Case study

Chris K felt very unwell, with constant tiredness, worsening memory and concentration, and little zest for life. He was depressed, had no sex drive and felt brain dead. His homocysteine score was 119. He changed his diet and took homocysteine-lowering nutrients and, within three months, his homocysteine level dropped to 19. After 6 months it had dropped to 11. He cannot believe how well he now feels. His memory and concentration are completely restored. He has boundless energy from 6 a.m. until 10 p.m. He now exercises for an hour every day and has lost weight. 'You have saved my life, or at least made it worth living again. I'm a new man and my love life has perked up,' says Chris.

Follow my H Factor Diet

A few years ago I devised the H Factor Diet – ten easy dietary changes that will help to lower your homocysteine level. Here they are.

1. **Eat less fatty meat, more fish and vegetable protein**
   Eat no more than four servings of lean meat a week; fish (not fried) at least three times a week; and if you're not allergic or intolerant, a serving of a soya-based food, such as tofu, tempeh or soya sausages, or beans, such as kidney beans, chickpea hummus or baked beans, at least five times a week.

2. **Eat your greens**
   Have at least five servings of fruit or vegetables a day. This means eating two pieces of fruit every single day, and three servings of vegetables. Vary your selections from day to day. Make sure half of what's on your plate for each main meal is vegetables.

3. **Have a clove of garlic a day**
   Either eat a clove of garlic a day, or take a garlic supplement every day. You can take garlic oil capsules or powdered garlic supplements.

4. **Don't add salt to your food**
   Don't add salt while you're cooking or to the food on your plate. The only salt I consider healthy is Solo salt, which has half the sodium of ordinary salt and lots of potassium and magnesium. Use this in moderation instead.

5. **Cut back on tea and coffee**
   Don't drink more than one cup of caffeinated or decaffeinated coffee, or two cups of tea, in a day. Instead choose from the wide variety of herbal teas and grain coffees available.

6. **Limit your alcohol**
   Limit your alcohol intake to no more than half a pint of beer, or one glass of red wine, in a day. Ideally, limit your intake to two pints of beer or four glasses of wine a week.

7. **Reduce your stress**
   If you are under a lot of stress, or find yourself reacting stressfully much of the time, make a decision to reduce your stress load by changing both the circumstances that are giving you stress and your attitude. Simple solutions abound: you can do yoga, meditation and/or exercise, or see a counsellor if you have some issues to resolve. These steps can make all the difference.

8. **Stop smoking**
   If you smoke, make a decision to stop, and seek help to do it. There is simply no safe level of smoking as far as homocysteine and your health is concerned. Smoking is nothing less than slow suicide. The sooner you stop the longer you'll live.

9. **Correct oestrogen deficiency**
   If you are postmenopausal, or have menopausal symptoms or other menstrual irregularities, check your oestrogen and progesterone levels with a hormone saliva test. If you are oestrogen or progesterone deficient, you can correct this with 'natural progesterone' HRT in the form of a transdermal skin cream. Natural progesterone has none of the associated risks of HRT, which include an increased risk for breast cancer, stroke and dementia.[74] From progesterone the body can make its own oestrogen if it needs to.

10. **Supplement a high-strength multivitamin every day**
    Excellent-quality multis are available in every health food store and some supermarkets. To keep your homocysteine levels in check, you'll need one that gives at least 25mg of B6, 200mcg of folic acid and 10mcg of B12. (See Resources, page 251, for suppliers.)

This diet, lifestyle and supplement plan has the potential to halve your homocysteine score in weeks. The goal is to bring your score to below 7. (Mine is 4.5.) Your homocysteine score is probably the best objective measure of whether you are achieving optimum nutrition for you.

Summary: keeping your homocysteine levels low

- Test your homocysteine level.
- If it's above 7, supplement the levels of homocysteine-lowering nutrients given in the table on page 97.
- Also take a high-strength multivitamin giving at least 25mg of B6, 200mcg of folic acid and 10mcg of B12, even if your H score isn't above 7.
- Follow the H Factor Diet shown in the preceding pages, eating plenty of greens and beans.
- Re-test yourself every three months until your homocysteine is below 7. Then test yourself once a year (see page 249 for test details).

Dig deeper by reading my book, co-authored with Dr James Braly, *The H Factor*. Also see www.thehfactor.com.

8

Antioxidant Protection

AGEING, BE IT OF THE brain or body, is what happens when the total load of environmental stresses and toxins you're exposed to lowers your capacity to adapt. In the previous chapter we learnt that there are two ways in which we lose cellular control, and succumb to Alzheimer's and other degenerative 21st-century diseases. One is faulty methylation, and the other is excess oxidation.

According to Professor Denham Harman from the University of Nebraska Medical School, there's a 99 per cent chance that free radicals are the basis for ageing. These oxidants, produced by the body every time we turn glucose into energy, eventually kill us. If we take in more oxidants, by smoking or living in a polluted city for example, and consume few antioxidants from fruit and vegetables, we age even more quickly.

So aside from avoiding pollutants such as cigarette and exhaust fumes whenever possible, antioxidants would seem to be key to holding brain degeneration at bay – and in this chapter we will explore how to get the best on offer. But first, let's look at the process of oxidation, the better to understand how antioxidants can disarm its effects.

A hundred thousand blows

To make energy we need glucose plus oxygen. Roughly a trillion molecules of oxygen are processed by each cell of the body each day. The free radicals generated by this process wound the cell's DNA – its genetic material – about 100,000 times. Antioxidants and our own immune system repair 99 per cent of the damage, but the rest continues to accumulate. According to geneticist Bruce Ames from the University of California, Berkeley, 'By the time you're old, we find a few million oxygen lesions per cell.'

What's more, we do seem to be programmed for obsolescence. Once men and women have passed their primary reproductive years, their ability to repair DNA damage declines and indeed, there is a strong association between this and the lifespan of any species. This lost ability to repair DNA is essentially a lost ability to adapt to our environment.

So, come the age of 50, unless you take positive steps to prevent it, your body will age rapidly. That's the bad news. The good news is that most if not all the scientists specialising in ageing, who are known as gerontologists, now agree that simple ways already exist to add at least 10, if not 20 years to your healthy lifespan. Here's what the experts say:

> Ultimately we are going to be able to get people to live a lot longer than anyone thinks.
> *Dr Bruce Ames, University of California researcher and geneticist*

> We could add an extra 12 to 18 years to our lives by taking 3200 to 12,000mg of vitamin C a day.
> *Dr Linus Pauling, twice Nobel Prize winner who put vitamin C on the map – and died at 92*

> Well-rounded nutrition, including generous amounts of vitamins C and E, can contribute materially to extending lifespan of those who are already middle-aged.
>
> *Dr Roger Williams, University of Austin, Texas, who helped discover folic acid and pantothenic acid – and died at 96*

As I asked earlier, however: what's the point of living longer if you can't remember your life? Well, the good news is that the right combination of antioxidants is an incredibly powerful protector of your memory.

The best vitamins for boosting your mood and memory are the antioxidants, which include the vitamins A, C and E, although the minerals selenium and zinc and the semi-essential nutrient co-enzyme Q10 have antioxidant properties too. These not only protect the brain from the insidious process of oxidation, but also improve the supply of oxygen, the brain's most crucial nutrient.

So too do B vitamins, especially folic acid and B12 – a deficiency of which results in anaemia and an inability to efficiently transport oxygen to the brain – and vitamins B1, B2 and B3, which help the brain use oxygen more efficiently and so generate energy. They do this in different ways: B1 acts as a co-enzyme in converting glucose into energy in muscles and nerves, including neurons; B2 is involved in regenerating the important antioxidant glutathione; and B3 acts as a co-factor in cell respiration, including that of neurons.

The more antioxidants you have in your blood, the sharper your mind. That's what researchers at the University of Berne in Switzerland found when they tested 442 people aged 65 to 94 years. Those with the highest levels of vitamin C and beta-carotene (the precursor to vitamin A found in plants) in their blood had the best scores on memory tests.[75] Other researchers in the US have found a similar positive link between vitamin E and memory performance.[76]

The likely explanation for these associations is that antioxidants improve circulation to the brain, and reduce the risk for vascular disease.[77] It is becoming more and more evident, as we saw earlier, that Alzheimer's and vascular disease share many of the same risk factors and mechanisms. As arteries become more and more inflamed and damaged, so too does the brain.

Antioxidants not only protect the brain from oxidation; they also reduce inflammation. The pain, redness or swelling that often result from inflammation are signals from the body letting you know something is wrong. Inflammation can happen, for instance, when the liver is overburdened (say, by binge drinking) and its capacity to detoxify is exceeded. Reducing inflammation is key to Alzheimer's prevention, as we've seen. So although you might not think of liver and brain in the same context, there is an interdependence here: improving liver function by increasing your intake of liver-friendly nutrients such as antioxidants, methylsulfonyl-methane or MSM, glutathione and cysteine helps lessen the burden on the brain.

Vitamins C and E protect your brain

Let's look more closely at how antioxidants – specifically vitamins C and E – keep your brain in top shape.

C and E are truly a dynamic duo when it comes to protecting your brain. First, vitamin E is fat-soluble, so it protects fatty tissue – and that's what most of the dry weight of your brain is made up of. Meanwhile, vitamin C is water-soluble, so it protects the rest (and with roughly three-quarters of your brain consisting of water, that's a lot). Vitamin C also recycles vitamin E and puts it back to work, after quenching a toxic oxidant. In the diagram overleaf you can see how oxidants damage the fatty acids that make up the membranes of neurons in the brain. Vitamin E is their bodyguard.

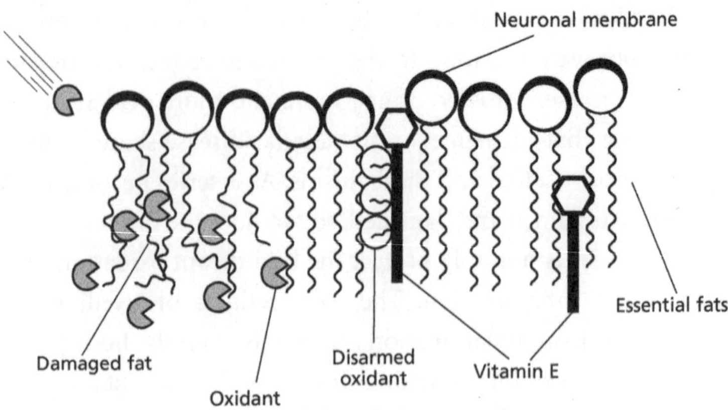

Figure 12. Oxidants damage fatty acids that make up neuronal membranes in the brain. Vitamin E protects these fatty acids from damage

By protecting the brain in this way, vitamin E not only plays a key role in early prevention of memory loss and dementia, but also in slowing down the progression of Alzheimer's. In a landmark study reported in the *New England Journal of Medicine* in 1997, Alzheimer's patients received either 2000ius of vitamin E, the drug Selegiline, or a placebo.[78] Vitamin E was shown to reduce progression most significantly, thus relieving some burden on both patients and their families. Another study in the US gave 633 disease-free 65–year-olds large amounts of either vitamin E or vitamin C. By the laws of probability a small number in each group would have been expected to show the signs of Alzheimer's five years later. None did.[79]

However, a more recent better-designed study failed to find a benefit for supplemental vitamin E versus placebo.[80] Other studies have reported a slower decline in memory in those combining antioxidants with medication.[81–2] There is also consistent evidence that the risk of developing Alzheimer's is lower in those with a high dietary intake of vitamin E and other antioxidants versus those with a low intake.[83–4]

By the way, not all forms of vitamin E are equal. Natural vitamin E, called d-alpha tocopherol, is 38 per cent more potent as an antioxidant than the synthetic dl-alpha tocopherol. There are also many kinds of tocopherols – alpha, beta, delta, gamma and so on. Recent research is highlighting the potential importance of gamma-tocopherol. Some vitamin E supplements provide d-alpha tocopherol in a blend of mixed tocopherols.

The power of synergy

In the last chapter we learnt how combining vitamins designed to lower homocysteine has a much more powerful effect than giving nutrients in isolation. It amazes me how this simple and factual principle of synergy is ignored in most research in nutrition today. A recent trial in 4,740 people over the age of 65 years illustrates the point clearly.[85]

This study, carried out in Cache County, Utah, followed up the participants over five years and identified over 200 cases of Alzheimer's disease. Those people who supplemented both vitamin E and vitamin C reduced their risk to a quarter of those who did not. Those who took vitamin E and a multivitamin also reduced their risk, but those who took either vitamin E on its own, or vitamin C on its own, did not.

Not all studies involving vitamin combinations have been positive, however. One large and well-designed study giving people with cardiovascular disease or diabetes a combination of 250mg of vitamin C, 600mg of synthetic vitamin E and 20mg of beta-carotene failed to find an improvement in cognitive function.[86] It is possible, however, that the forms and amounts of vitamins given to these already sick people just weren't enough to reduce oxidation. Unfortunately, the researchers didn't measure oxidative stress, so we'll never know.

The moral of the story is to take the right combination, and the right dose of antioxidant nutrients. The diagram below shows you the main antioxidant team players – vitamin E, vitamin C, beta-carotene, glutathione, anthocyanidins, lipoic acid and co-enzyme Q10 – and how they work together to disarm a brain-damaging oxidant.

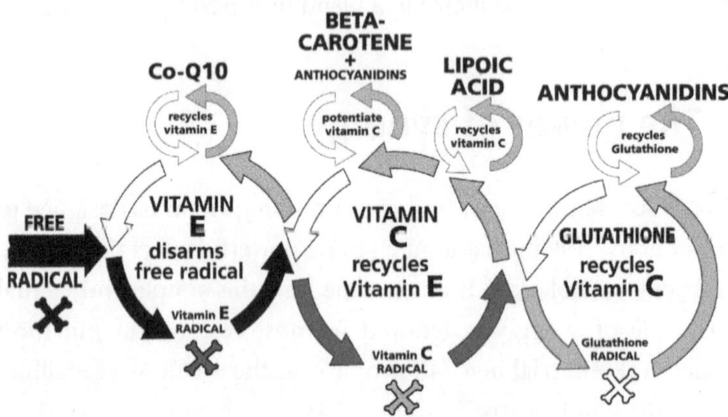

Figure 13. A fat-based oxidant, technically called a free radical, can be disarmed by vitamin E. The vitamin E molecule then becomes a free radical. It is effectively recycled and put back to work by vitamin C and Co-Q10. In turn, vitamin C is recycled by glutathione, lipoic acid and beta-carotene. Glutathione is recycled by anthocyanidins including resveratrol

While most multis give you small amounts of these antioxidants, there's a good case for upping your intake as you get older. For vitamin C, I recommend as an optimum amount 1g, plus an additional gram for every two decades above 40. So, if you are 40 plus, take 2g; if you're 60 plus, take 3g; and if you're 80 plus, take 4g. Vitamin C is water soluble and enters and leaves the body within four to six hours, so take it in divided doses. If you're taking 3g a day, for example, have 1g with each meal.

For vitamin E the magic formula is 200mg up to age 40, then add 100mg per decade, making 300mg when you are 40, 400mg when you are 50, and 500mg when you are 60 or above.

Practically speaking, the best way to do all this is to start with a high-strength multivitamin and 2 additional grams of vitamin C, then add an 'antioxidant complex' from the age of 40, then add some additional vitamin E and C as you get older, or take more of the antioxidant complex. Complicated as that advice might sound, I'm going to make it dead easy for you in Part 3.

Increase your dietary antioxidants

As important as supplements are, they are just that – a supplement to your diet. No supplement will give you the all-round antioxidant protection that you'll get from literally hundreds of antioxidants in foods.

The main essential antioxidant vitamins are A, C and E and the precursor of vitamin A, beta-carotene. Beta-carotene is found in red, orange and yellow vegetables and fruit. Vitamin C is also abundant in vegetables and fruit eaten raw, but heat rapidly destroys it. Vitamin E is found in 'seed' foods, including nuts, seeds and their oils, and vegetables like peas, broad beans, corn and whole grains.

However, there are many other important antioxidant ingredients in food. Examples are quercitin in onions, catechins in green tea, epicatechin in chocolate, isoflavones in beans, and anthocyanidins, including resveratrol in berries and red grapes. The more of these you eat the lower your risk of memory decline.[87] It's far better to eat a varied diet high in antioxidant-rich foods than to simply rely on vitamin C and E. Thanks to research at Tufts University in Boston, there's a way to rate a food's overall antioxidant power. Each food can now be assigned a certain number of ORAC (short for 'oxygen radical absorbance capacity') units. Foods that score high in these units are especially helpful in countering free-radical damage in your body.

My top 20 foods are shown in the table overleaf. Each of these food servings gives you 2,000 ORACs. If you can, eat the equivalent of 6,000 ORACs a day. The more ORACs you take in the more you protect your memory.[88] You'll also be better protected against many diseases, including cancer and heart disease.

The chart below shows the ORAC units of twenty different foods that you can incorporate easily into your daily diet. Each serving contains approximately 2,000 units. Just pick at least three of these daily to hit your target of 6,000.

1 ⅓ tsp cinnamon, ground
2 ½ tsp oregano, dried
3 ½ tsp turmeric, ground
4 1 heaped tsp mustard
5 ⅕ cup blueberries
6 ½ a pear, grapefruit or plum
7 ½ cup blackcurrants & berries, raspberries, strawberries
8 ½ cup cherries or a shot of CherryActive concentrate
9 An orange or apple
10 4 pieces of dark chocolate (70% cocoa)
11 7 walnut halves
12 8 pecan halves
13 ¼ cup pistachios
14 ½ cup cooked lentils
15 1 cup cooked kidney beans
16 ⅓ medium avocado
17 ½ cup of red cabbage
18 2 cups of broccoli
19 1 medium artichoke or 8 spears of asparagus
20 1 medium glass (150ml) red wine

Source: Oxygen Radical Absorbance Capacity of Selected Foods – 2007, US Department of Agriculture

Generally speaking, where you find the most colour and flavour you will also find the highest antioxidant levels. The reds, yellows and oranges of tomatoes and carrots, for example are due to the presence of beta-carotene. Artichoke has the highest rating of vegetables whereas other vegetables, such as carrots, peas and spinach are lower in units, so aim for five to ten servings daily of a range of fruits and vegetables to keep your intake high.

Fruits that have the highest levels are those with the deepest colour, such as blueberries, raspberries and strawberries. These are particularly rich in powerful antioxidants called anthocyanadins. One cup of blueberries will provide 9,697 units. You would need to eat 11 bananas to get the same benefit as a cupful of blueberries!

One of the simplest and easiest ways to achieve 6,000 ORACs is to have a daily shot of a montmorency cherry concentrate called CherryActive, diluted with water. This measures 8,260 on the ORAC scale, which is the equivalent of around 23 portions of regular fruit and vegetables! Other juices claim high ORAC scores, from acai to pomegranate, but this tops the lot.

Not just any 'five a day'

The number of portions of fruit and vegetables you need per day really does depend on your choices, as you can see in the two day's menus below. Both days have five portions selected, but Day 2's selection is 8,000 ORACs more than Day 1's.

Day 1		Day 2	
Fruit/Vegetable portion	**ORAC**	**Fruit/Vegetable portion**	**ORAC**
⅛ large cantaloupe melon	315	Half a pear	2617
Kiwi fruit	802	Half a cup of strawberries	2683
1 medium carrot, raw	406	Half an avocado	2899
½ cup green peas, frozen	432	1 cup broccoli, raw	1226
1 cup spinach, raw	455	4 spears asparagus, boiled	986
Total Score	2410	Total Score	10411

A good example of an antioxidant-rich diet is a Mediterranean diet, which is also associated with reduced risk for

Alzheimer's.[89] It appears to be that a higher intake of fruit, vegetables and fish decreases risk while a higher intake of meat and dairy products increases risk. Other studies have shown that those who consume either more fruit and vegetables, or more tea, chocolate or red wine tend to have better cognition.[90]

As you can see from the chart, the best fruit are berries. Another great antioxidant fruit is watermelon. The flesh is high in beta-carotene and vitamin C, while the seeds are high in vitamin E and in the antioxidant minerals zinc and selenium.You can make a great antioxidant cocktail by removing the rind on a chunk of it and putting it into the blender, seeds and all. Seeds and seafood are the best all-round dietary sources of selenium and zinc.

The amino acids cysteine and glutathione act as antioxidants. They help make one of the body's key antioxidant enzymes, glutathione peroxidase, which is itself dependent on selenium. This enzyme helps to detoxify the body, protecting us against exhaust fumes, carcinogens, infections, too much alcohol and toxic metals. Cysteine and glutathione are particularly abundant in white meat, tuna, lentils, beans, nuts, seeds, onions and garlic, and have been shown to boost the immune system as well as increase antioxidant power.

Can red wine or resveratrol protect your mind?

A number of studies have found a link between a higher intake of the antioxidant resveratrol, found in red wine, and reduced risk of memory decline.[91] This has led to animal studies that have shown that supplementing resveratrol leads to less formation of plaques in the brain, as seen in Alzheimer's.[92] It's too soon to extrapolate this to us humans but if you do choose to take an all-round antioxidant supplement this is certainly a nutrient I'd consider taking. The ideal amount to supplement is 20mg a day. A glass of merlot may give you 2 to 4mg.

Summary: minimising oxidation, maximising antioxidants

- Don't smoke, and minimise the time you spend in smoky and polluted places.
- Try to avoid eating deep-fried food. Poach, steam or steam-fry food instead.
- Eat half your diet raw or lightly steamed.
- Have six or more servings of fruit and vegetables a day, emphasising high-ORAC fruits, vegetables, herbs and spices (aim for 6,000 ORACs a day).
- Snack on fresh fruit.
- Supplement at least 1g of vitamin C, plus 400mg of vitamin E and 20mg of beta-carotene a day.
- Ideally, also take an all-round antioxidant supplement formula containing either glutathione or N-acetyl cysteine, co-enzyme Q10, lipoic acid, resveratrol, plus vitamins A, C and E.

9

Other Memory-boosting Vitamins, Minerals and Amino Acids

AS MENTIONED IN the last chapter, inflammation is the body's way of telling us something is out of kilter and in fact, it's an underlying cause of many of the diseases of later life – cancer, heart disease, diabetes and Alzheimer's. Increases in underlying inflammatory processes in the brain, which can ultimately lead to neuronal damage, can also leave our grey matter in dire need of certain nutrients.

Antioxidants aren't the only heroes in this story. Here are the best of the rest:

- B vitamins
- Trace elements
- Essential fats
- Phospholipids.

We'll look at the first two on that list in this chapter, and the rest in subsequent chapters.

But can't we just get these goodies from a well-balanced diet?

Unfortunately, this is a misconception – and one that becomes increasingly further from the truth as you age. First, the ability of many people to digest and absorb nutrients decreases. A common finding among older people is that hydrochloric acid production in the stomach declines, immediately affecting their ability to make use of protein, vitamins and minerals. Many of us become less physically active as we age, too, and so end up losing our appetites, eating less – and thus taking in fewer nutrients. Circulation can also worsen with age, allowing fewer nutrients to make it from the gut to the brain.

And getting those nutrients into the brain is of paramount importance. While Part 1 gave you the background to the general importance to brain health of the 'famous five' (antioxidants, plus the four in the list opposite), they really come into their own in later life, as I have shown in this book. Most studies have not found a strong effect but perhaps the reason is because the usual multivitamin tablet contains doses of individual vitamins that are close to or below the RDA. In the opinion of eminent scientists such as Professor Bruce Ames at the University of California, there is a good reason for giving higher doses of multivitamin and mineral supplements based on optimal levels.

The most interesting result reported so far is in the pilot study involving 225 Alzheimer's patients who had not been on either medication or supplementation. They were given either placebos or a nutrient cocktail containing a combination of high-dose essential fats (300mg of EPA and 1200mg of DHA), phospholipids (400mg of choline – see chapter 11), antioxidants (40mg of vitamin E, 60mg of vitamin C and 60mcg of selenium), B vitamins (400mcg of folic acid, 3,000mcg of B12 and 1mg of B6) and uridine, which is a substance produced by the body that enhances synaptic growth.

This rather short 12–week trial showed clear improvements in memory for the patients taking the nutrient cocktail. These improvements were not seen in the placebo group. This is encouraging and paves the way for longer trials. The choice of nutrients also makes sense in that DHA is the main omega 3 fat that builds the brain, and phospholipids can be created in the brain, a process which is very dependent on methylation. Vitamin B6, folic acid and B12 are required for proper methylation and the elderly are often unable to absorb B12, hence the need for very high doses.[93]

But supplements don't just improve your mental performance; they also make you happier. Another double-blind placebo-controlled trial, for instance, gave elderly people a B complex supplement containing 10mg of B1, B2 and B6. (That's about 10 times the RDA.) Compared to those taking placebos, there was a definite improvement in mood.[94] This isn't just a good effect in itself. Many elderly people, particularly those suffering from cognitive decline, are also depressed – and depression can involve mental 'fogs' and exhaustion, which can exacerbate difficulties with cognition. So improving mood can also help get your mind into gear.

Those fabulous Bs

B vitamins do far more for the brain than simply reduce homocysteine levels (see Chapter 7). Oxygen, the most crucial – and dangerous – nutrient of them all, depends on vitamin B12, folic acid, niacin and essential fats to be transported and used by the brain, for instance. And it has long been known that vitamin B1 deficiency results in brain damage.

In fact, one of the most dangerous problems of excessive alcohol consumption is induced B1 deficiency – a condition called Wernicke-Korsakoff syndrome. The symptoms include anxiety and depression, obsessive thinking, confusion, defective memory (especially of recent events) and time distortion – which are not so different from Alzheimer's.

Vitamin B3 (niacin) is crucial for oxygen utilisation. It is incorporated into the co-enzyme NAD (nicotinamide adenosine dinucleotide), and many reactions involving oxygen need NAD. Without it, pellagra (a deficiency disease characterised by dermatitis, diarrhoea and dementia) and senility can develop. For these reasons, optimal intakes of all the B vitamins are an important part of an Alzheimer's prevention plan.

Why niacin keeps your mind sharp

Martha Morris of the Rush Institute for Healthy Aging at the US Centers for Disease Control and Prevention in Atlanta, Georgia, examined whether dietary intake of niacin was associated with Alzheimer's disease and cognitive decline. This study was conducted between 1993 and 2002 in a Chicago community of 6,158 residents aged 65 years and older.

Levels of niacin intake were determined by questionnaires, and cognitive tests were administered to all study participants twice over a six-year follow-up period. Clinical evaluations were performed on study participants initially unaffected by dementia, and 131 participants were diagnosed with Alzheimer's over the time of the study.

What the study found was that the higher a person's intake of niacin from their diet, the slower their annual rate of cognitive decline was. In fact, eating abundant amounts of niacin-rich foods increased protection against mental decline by 80 per cent. The researcher's conclusion was that 'dietary niacin may protect against Alzheimer's disease and age-related cognitive decline'.[95]

How does niacin manage it? It may be because niacin, or nicotinic acid, is thought to improve circulation, and the circulation of oxygen and nutrients in the brain are essential for it to function. Because of its effect on the circulation, however, niacin can make you blush if you have more than 30mg a day, especially on an empty stomach.

This blushing shouldn't be viewed as an adverse reaction, and if you take niacin with food, and on a regular basis, the blushing effect is reduced. Another form of vitamin B3, niacinamide, does not cause blushing, and thus may not be so effective at stimulating circulation. It is certainly not as effective in lowering cholesterol, which is another positive side-effect of niacin. You can take 'no-flush' niacin (inositol hexanicotinate), which both lowers cholesterol and is good for the mind. My advice, if you wish to add niacin to your brain-boosting programme, is to take 100mg of niacin or no-flush niacin a day in addition to whatever is in your multivitamin.

Amino acid stars

Acetyl-l-carnitine

The amino acid acetyl-l-carnitine, or ALC for short, is an important factor in promoting healthy brain function, memory and neurotransmitter production. ALC is derived from the amino acids methionine and lysine and is commonly found in foods such as beef, lamb, vegetables and grains. It is widely available in supplement form, frequently in combination with lipoic acid (see opposite).

It acts as a powerful antioxidant within the brain cell, stabilises cell membranes, improves energy production within the brain cell, and enhances or mimics the function of the memory neurotransmitter, acetylcholine. In fact, along with choline, ALC is a key co-factor in acetylcholine production. And as this neurotransmitter helps to control memory, attention and cognitive functions such as awareness, perception, reasoning and judgement, that is a very important task.

It has been found that in people who already have Alzheimer's and dementia, supplementing ALC has a very positive effect on mental function. In one study conducted over the period of one year, Alzheimer's patients taking ALC showed a slower rate of mental decline, suggesting that it actually helps to slow the progression of the disease.[96] ALC has also been shown to reduce blood cortisol levels,[97] which is vital given the negative effects of this stress hormone on the brain (more on this in Chapter 14). Another study involving elderly patients over a period of five months showed significant improvement in learning, memory and 'negative feelings' during and after supplementation with ALC.[98]

A number of studies have shown significant improvement in learning and memory in rats, particularly when ALC is given in combination with lipoic acid.[99–100] (Lipoic acid is a potent antioxidant found in foods such as spinach, liver, and brewer's yeast.) This study found that the animals given the supplements also had younger-looking brains, with less neuronal damage. More thorough clinical trials are needed to confirm any effects of ALC in preventing or treating Alzheimer's disease.

Glutamine

Since we know that the amino acid glutamine is converted into the neurotransmitter GABA (see page 42) in the brain, could supplementing glutamine also help memory? In fact, a Chinese study showed just that – that glutamine supplementation improved the learning ability and memory of rats.[101–2] Another team of researchers at the University of Utah studied the brain levels of GABA in a group of very old macaque monkeys. They found that the oldest monkeys had the lowest levels of GABA in the brain. By giving the monkeys GABA, their mental agility improved by two to three times over.[103]

Summary: getting enough extra vitamins, minerals and amino acids

- Take a high strength all-round multivitamin every day.
- Supplement 100mg of niacin daily, with food.
- Supplement 250mg of acetyl-l-carnitine and 120mg of lipoic acid.
- Supplement 1g of L-glutamine. This is available as a tablet and as a powder that dissolves in water (take the equivalent of 1g, half a teaspoon, in water on an empty stomach).

10

Fats That Make You Think Faster

IF YOU TAKE OUT all the water from your brain, most of the rest of it is fat – 60 per cent, in fact. This fatty tissue needs replenishing, but not with just any old fat. Some fats are not only positively good for you, they are absolutely vital for mental health. Not only do you need them to stay free from age-related memory decline; you also need them in optimal amounts if you want to maximise your intelligence. This is the chapter where we'll find out how to make that a reality.

Our ability to make our way successfully through life depends upon a balance of mental, emotional and physical intelligence. Mental intelligence we are well aware of, with IQ tests that determine a person's ability to make intellectual connections and deal with complex concepts. But emotional intelligence is no less important. Your 'EQ' is a measure of your ability to respond emotionally to situations in an appropriate and sensitive way. If you lose your temper easily, and oscillate between depression and hyperactivity, lacking emotional balance and perspective, there's room for improvement, however 'bright' you are.

Then there's physical intelligence. Your 'PQ' is all about your brain–body coordination. It's known, for instance, that we become less physically coordinated the more we're in the grip of age-related memory loss or dementia.

Each type of intelligence is affected by our intake of the so-called essential fats, the omega-3s and omega-6s.

The crucial fats

Conclusive research now clearly shows that the type of fat you eat, as well as the amount, has a profound effect on how you think and feel. This is down to the simple fact that the brain and nervous system are totally dependent on a group of fats. These include:

- Saturated and monounsaturated fat
- Cholesterol
- Omega-3 (polyunsaturated) fat – especially EPA and DHA
- Omega-6 (polyunsaturated) fat – especially GLA and AA.

As we learnt in Chapter 6, the first two types of fat can be made in the body, so we won't concentrate on them here. The omega fats, however, have to be topped up through diet.

To understand why these fats are so important, let's take a closer look at a brain cell. If you recall from Chapter 2, the making of intelligence involves the careful connecting up of billions of nerve cells, each one of which links to as many as 20,000 others. The 'messengers', neurotransmitters, deliver their messages across connection points called synapses into receptor sites. These receptor sites are contained within a sheath made of myelin. This substance is a bit like a layer of insulation around an electrical wire and is roughly 75 per cent fat. But what kind of fat?

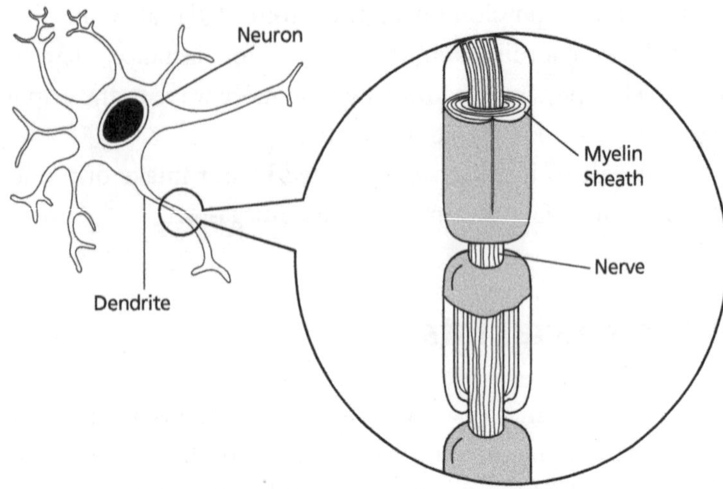

Figure 14. The myelin sheath surrounding nerves is made out of phospholipids and essential fats

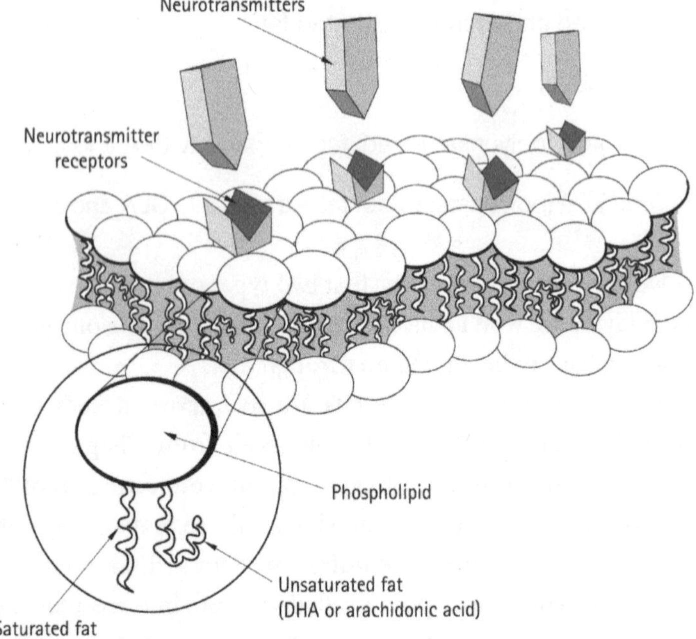

Figure 15. Phospholipids have two kinds of fatty acids attached – a saturated and an unsaturated fatty acid. The former gives solidity and the latter, flexibility

The myelin sheath is made out of phospholipids (more on these in the next chapter) that each have a saturated and unsaturated fatty acid attached (see figure opposite). The unsaturated fatty acid (bent) is usually an omega-3 fat called DHA or an omega-6 fat called arachidonic acid. This arrangement of fats seems to be the crucial one for the brain's structure and function. So for brain health, both omega-3 and omega-6 fat families must be present in your diet. If you answered 'yes' to more than four questions in the Essential Fat Check on page 61, the chances are you are deficient.

Ocean riches

The first evidence for the vital role essential fats play in the brain emerged when the difference in Alzheimer's risk between fish eaters and non-fish eaters was examined. A study by Dr Martha Morris and colleagues from Chicago's Rush Institute for Healthy Aging found that eating fish once a week can slash your risk of developing Alzheimer's by as much as 60 per cent. Their study followed 815 people, aged 65 to 94 years, for seven years, and found that dietary intake of fish was strongly linked to Alzheimer's risk. They found that the strongest link was the amount of DHA, a form of omega-3 fat found in oily, cold water, carnivorous fish such as mackerel and salmon. The higher a person's dietary intake of DHA, the lower their risk of developing Alzheimer's.[104]

Another study found that people who regularly consumed omega-3 rich oils, such as canola oil, flaxseed oil and walnut oil, reduced their risk of dementia by 60 per cent compared to people who did not regularly consume such oils. People who ate fruits and vegetables daily also reduced their risk of dementia by 30 per cent compared to those who didn't regularly eat fruits and vegetables.

The study also found people who ate fish at least once a week had a 35 per cent lower risk of Alzheimer's disease and 40 per cent lower risk of dementia, but only if they did not carry the gene that increases the risk of Alzheimer's, called apolipoprotein E4, or ApoE4. As the researchers said, 'Given that most people do not carry the ApoE4 gene, these results could have considerable implications in terms of public health.'[105]

DHA, along with EPA, are the two most powerful omega-3 fats. EPA is more 'functional' in the brain – for example, it enhances serotonin levels and consequently mood. EPA has also been shown to help with depression, manic depression and schizophrenia more effectively than DHA. DHA, however, is thought to have more of a structural role and is needed to build brain cells.

Until recently, little was known about the benefits of omega-3 DHA fish oil supplements in adults. A study, conducted by a clinical research department in Columbia, involved 485 participants over the age of 55 who were showing signs of memory decline but were otherwise considered as healthy.[106] After taking DHA, positive improvements were shown. A further study – involving 402 individuals with mild Alzheimer's given DHA over an 18-month period – didn't show improvements, perhaps indicating that it is too late in the disease process.[107]

The latest study, carried out at Massey University in New Zealand, tested 176 adults between the ages of 18 and 45 who ate fish infrequently. The participants were given 1,160 mg of omega-3 DHA fish oil supplements or a placebo over a six-month period. Each participant went through a cognitive function and reaction test before and after the study. Those who took the DHA supplement showed significant improvements in their episodic (ability to recall past personal events at a particular time) and working memory (ability to execute verbal and non-verbal tasks) and an improvement in their reaction time.[108]

The amount given in these studies was quite high and equates to eating the equivalent of a serving of oily fish almost every day. While this might not appear practical, having three servings of oily fish a week, a serving of cod roe or taramaslata and supplementing 250mg of DHA a day would give you about 1,000mg a day. Whether lower doses would produce the same effect will not be known until more studies are carried out.

Fish for the Brain

While much attention has been focused on the omega-3 fats in fish, many studies have found an improvement in mental health, and a decreased risk of Alzheimer's, in those eating more fish in general, not just oily fish. Analysis of the data from the Hoordland health survey indicates that the more fish you eat, up to a maximum of 75g per day, which is a small serving, the better your memory and mental health. A number of studies have found that total fish intake is actually a much better predictor of low risk for dementia than intake of omega-3 fats such as EPA and DHA.[109] While high meat consumption tends to increase risk, it suggests that something in fish other than protein or essential fats is delivering a health benefit. Fish is also an excellent source of B12, as well as niacin (B3), which is a known memory booster. It's also an excellent source of the antioxidants selenium and zinc. Fish is also one of the best sources of choline which, as you'll discover in the next chapter, is vital for brain function. In addition, it is very rich in vitamin D.

Vitamin D

Vitamin D is a fat-based vitamin that acts more like a hormone. It is made in the skin from the action of sunlight on cholesterol. The further away from the Equator you live, and the less you expose yourself to natural light, the less you make. The survival of those in the far North, for example the Inuit, is dependent on a diet containing the oily fish that store this vitamin.

While it used to be thought that vitamin D was only necessary for bone health, in recent years it has become very clear that vitamin D is vital for the immune system and for mental health – and that most people in Britain don't get enough. For example, many consider the optimal intake of vitamin D is a blood level of 75 µmol/l or more. During the winter only 13 per cent of British adults achieve this.[110] This is especially relevant since the lower your vitamin D the greater your risk of Alzheimer's.[111] Vitamin D is known to affect the brain in ways that could be of benefit in memory protection,[112] although good clinical trials are yet to be performed.

Ideally you need to take in about 30mcg of vitamin D a day. Oily fish are by far the best source (a 100g serving of mackerel will give you 8mcg). There is a little in eggs (about 1mcg). This means that if you ate three servings of oily fish a week and six eggs you'd be averaging about 4mcg a day. If you also get outside for half an hour a day and expose some of your skin to sunlight you might possibly achieve an average of 15mcg a day (obviously more in the summer or in a hot country). So I think it is well worth supplementing 15mcg a day. Better multivitamins contain this much. The RDA, which is out of date, is only 5mcg.

Coconut oil

Of growing interest is the use of organic cold-pressed coconut oil or butter, which is a different type of saturated fat called a medium chain triglyceride (MCT). The liver turns MCTs into ketones, an alternative energy source for neurons, which, in the same way hybrid cars can burn two fuels, can burn glucose or ketones. There's a lot of evidence of sugar problems in Alzheimer's, so cells might be unable to use it properly as a fuel. With plenty of anecdotal reports of amazing and immediate improvement in patients given 35 grams of coconut oil a day – possibly because cells are able to use MCTs properly as fuel – it certainly warrants a controlled trial. Switching dysfunctional brain cells to run on ketones could give a big energy and memory boost, but it is less likely that this itself would prevent the actual neuronal degeneration, although it might slow it down.

How to get the best fats

While the research on omega-3 fish oils is under way, it's worth upping your intake of essential fats, especially omega-3s, by eating three servings of oily fish (herring, wild or organic salmon, mackerel or fresh tuna) a week. This simple strategy is already known to halve your risk of a heart attack, and cardiovascular disease and memory decline are intimately connected.

Omega-3 fats are not only extremely powerful anti-inflammatory agents – and don't forget that inflammation is one of the main ways brain cells get damaged – but they may also be involved in encoding memories. One theory is that memories are encoded in lipoproteins, built out of essential fats and phospholipids. Another is that memories are encoded through RNA, the messenger molecule in charge of building new cells. This seems plausible: as brain cells are permanently being replaced and rebuilt, memory must be transmittable. If this theory is correct, zinc is a key to memory because it is essential for building RNA. And fish is not only a good source of omega-3 fats, it's also rich in both RNA and zinc.

There are three ways to up your intake of essential fats: eat seeds and fish; eat seed oils, which have a higher concentration of essential fats but don't provide other nutrients which are abundant in the whole seeds; or supplement concentrated fish oils and seed oils such as flax, evening primrose or starflower oil.

Seed oils

If you want to go for oils, the best place to start is an oil blend that offers a 1:1 ratio of omega-3 and omega-6 fats. You want an oil blend that is cold-pressed, preferably organic and kept refrigerated before you buy it. These are now widely available in health food stores. You need about a dessertspoon a day of such an oil, and can add it to salads and other foods (without heating) or just take it neat. Hemp seed oil is the next best thing. It provides 19 per cent alpha-linolenic acid (an omega-3), 57 per cent linoleic acid and 2 per cent GLA (both omega-6).

Essential fat supplements

As far as supplements are concerned, for omega-6 your best bet is starflower (borage) oil or evening primrose oil. Starflower oil provides more GLA and you need at least 100mg of GLA a day. Fish oils are best for omega-3 and you need at least 400mg of EPA and 400mg of DHA. So, either supplement one GLA capsule and however many fish oil capsules rich in EPA and DHA it takes to reach 400mg of each, or find a supplement that combines EPA, DHA and GLA in the appropriate amounts, and take two a day.

These levels of essential fats promote brain function and health. The quantities should be doubled if you scored high on the Essential Fat Check (see page 61), until your symptoms go away. (If you have a problem that responds well to essential fats, such as depression, you may even need more. This is explained in my book, *Optimum Nutrition for the Mind*.)

Summary: ensuring you get enough brain fats

- Eat seeds and nuts – the best seeds are chia, flax, hemp, pumpkin, sunflower and sesame. You get more goodness out of them by grinding them first and sprinkling on cereal, soups and salads.

- Eat coldwater carnivorous fish – a serving of herring, mackerel, wild or organic salmon or fresh tuna two or three times a week provides a good source of omega-3 fats.
- Use cold-pressed seed oils – either choose an oil blend or hemp oil for salad dressings and other uses not involving heat, such as drizzling on vegetables.
- Minimise your intake of fried food, processed food and saturated fat from meat and dairy products.
- Supplement fish oil for omega-3 fats and starflower or evening primrose oil for omega-6 fats. Once you hit the age of 50, I recommend 1000mg of combined DHA/EPA a day. With a supplement providing 400 to 600mg, this means two fish oil capsules a day. Since DHA appears the most important, make sure you are getting at least 400mg of this.

In practical terms, you may want to pursue a combined strategy to ensure an optimal intake of brain fats. Here's what I recommend:

- A tablespoon of ground seeds – most days.
- Cold-pressed seed oil blend – on salad dressings and on vegetables.
- Coldwater carnivorous fish – twice a week (but limit tuna to three times a month).
- EPA/DHA/GLA supplement – once a day.

Also, make sure you supplement 10mcg of vitamin D a day, and get some exposure to natural light every day.

11

Phospholipids – The Vital Brain Builders

THERE'S ANOTHER FAMILY of fats that is just as important for the smooth working of your brain as the omegas: phospholipids. We've already encountered these 'smart' fats several times. Now let's get the full lowdown on what they do, and how to get an adequate supply.

Phospholipids have turned out to be essential in animals, and are almost certainly essential in humans, but they haven't been granted that official title yet. The reason? 'Essential' fats are called that because our bodies cannot make them, so we must ensure they're part of our diet; but the body can make phospholipids. The problem is, it doesn't make enough, so you still need to top them up. The best food sources are eggs, organ meats and brains – but those body bits don't grace many plates these days, and many people now mistakenly avoid eggs. The net result is a phospholipid deficiency for far too many of us.

In Chapter 10 we saw how important phospholipids are in keeping messages – which are actually neurotransmitters – flowing smoothly through the brain. That's because they're the insulation experts, helping make up the myelin sheath that not only protects all nerves (see page 122), but also speeds the transmission of messages between them. There are a number of different kinds of phospholipids, but the two main players are phosphatidyl choline and phosphatidyl serine. Not only do phospholipids enhance your mood, mind and mental performance, they also protect against age-related memory decline and Alzheimer's disease. This is because they have three essential roles in keeping your brain healthy:

- They're one of the brain's main construction materials
- Acetylcholine, the memory neurotransmitter, is built from choline (the most useable form of which is phosphatidyl choline)
- They help improve methylation and keep your homocysteine level low.

Acetylcholine: the memory molecule

A memory is not held in one, but in several brain cells joined together in a network. The memory itself is thought to be put into storage by the neurotransmitter acetylcholine, and stored by altering the structure of RNA – a molecule important in transcribing genetic information – within brain cells. The limbic system, the doughnut-shaped part of the brain that sits on top of the brain stem and is associated with emotion and motivation, then has to decide if the memory is worth keeping. A part of the limbic system known as the amygdala is involved in decisions about more emotional memories, while the hippocampus decides about others.

In Alzheimer's, the hippocampus loses its ability to file memories, resulting in an inability to create new ones. People with Alzheimer's also show marked deficiencies in acetylcholine, no doubt largely because acetylcholine-producing brain cells have been damaged or destroyed. Even if a memory is intact, if you don't have enough acetylcholine you can't connect one part of the memory with others. For example, you know the face but can't remember the name.

Acetylcholine is so important for memory that the leading drugs for dementia and Alzheimer's, such as Aricept (see Appendix 4, page 218), are based on boosting acetylcholine. They do this by blocking the enzyme that would normally break down acetylcholine, called acetylcholinesterase. These drugs, known as acetylcholinesterase inhibitors, therefore interfere with a normal process in the body, leading at most to a short-term benefit. They do nothing to correct any of the known underlying causes that lead to neuronal damage or falling acetylcholine levels. Providing the brain with essential nutrients such as phospholipids, essential fats and B vitamins makes more sense.

Acetylcholine is directly built from the nutrient choline, the most useable form of which is phosphatidyl choline. This phospholipid also helps to make membranes in the brain and therefore protect against a decline in numbers and efficiency of neurons. We tend to lose neurons and synapses as we age, which is why both memory and emotion become blunted. However, this doesn't need to happen if you can just get these phospholipids and essential fats into the brain.

As you can see from the figure opposite, what you want is to get choline into the brain. One way to do this is to supplement phosphatidyl choline directly. Or you can supplement DMAE (see page 136), which is the precursor for phosphatidyl choline. Since the phospholipids literally soak up essential fats – they're made up of one phosphorus-containing molecule such as choline, and two essential fatty acids – combining phosphatidyl choline with essential fats is like oysters for your brain. These can help keep you as sharp as a pencil throughout life.

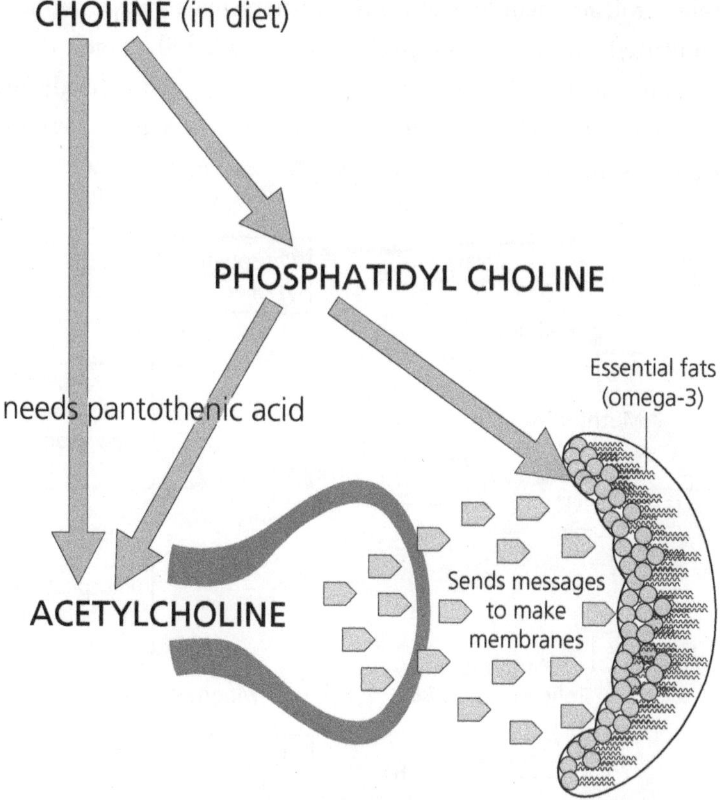

Figure 16. How the brain makes phospholipids and acetylcholine

How phospholipids keep homocysteine in check

As well as being the critical building blocks for your neurons, and the raw material from which the brain makes acetylcholine, phosphatidyl choline is an important nutrient for keeping your homocysteine level in check and for helping you stay 'well methylated' (see page 80). This is because choline contains three 'methyl' groups needed for the vital process of methylation, which is how the body and brain keeps thousands of critical biochemicals, including neurotransmitters, in balance. Choline is converted into trimethylglycine (also called 'betaine', as in 'betaine hydrochloride' or stomach acid), trimethylglycine donates a methyl group to homocysteine, and homocysteine becomes the vital brain nutrient SAMe (see Figure below).

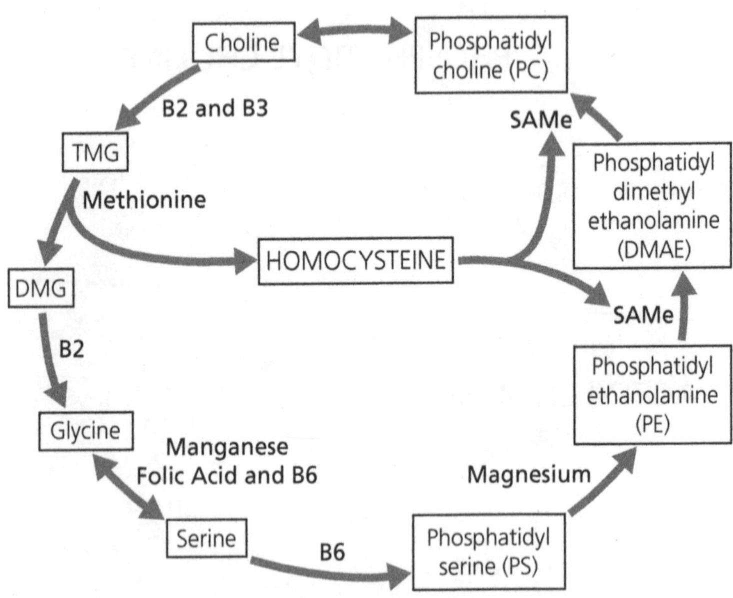

Figure 17. The Phospholipid Loop. The brain is made out of phospholipids – such as phosphatidyl choline, phosphatidyl ethanolamine and phosphatidyl serine. These are made from nutrients such as choline, rich in eggs, or DMAE, rich in fish. Their production depends on a number of vitamins and minerals, and especially B vitamins that help methylation, turning homocysteine into SAMe (s-adenosyl methionine)

SAMe then helps to turn one phospholipid into another, making sure that your brain has a second-by-second supply of all the building materials it needs to help keep its cells healthy.

Now that you know how phospholipids work to keep your brain healthy, let's look at the evidence that eating foods rich in phospholipids, or supplementing them, can help you keep your marbles and prevent a slide into dementia.

Potent PC (phosphatidyl choline)

One of the studies that really shows the potential power of phosphatidyl choline, a nutrient I supplement every day, was conducted by scientists at Duke University Medical Center in the US. They demonstrated that giving choline during pregnancy creates the equivalent of superbrains in the offspring.

The researchers fed some pregnant rats choline halfway through their pregnancy. The infant rats whose mothers were given choline had vastly superior brains with more neuronal connections, and consequently, improved learning ability and better memory recall, all of which persisted into old age. This research showed that giving choline helps restructure the brain for improved performance.[113]

No such study has been carried out on pregnant women and their babies so we can't automatically assume the same applies to humans. But having said that, I'd certainly recommend a pregnant woman to have a spoonful of lecithin granules or a lecithin capsule (one of the best sources of phosphatidyl choline) a day.

But what about the effects on memory in adults, and in people who already have Alzheimer's disease? After all, supplementing choline not only makes more acetylcholine,[114] the memory neurotransmitter; it is also a vital building material for nerve cells and the receptor sites for neurotransmitters. According to Professor Richard Wurtman of the Massachusetts Institute of Technology (MIT), if your choline levels are depleted, your body grabs the choline you need to build your nerve cells to make more acetylcholine.[115] So, Wurtman believes, providing the brain with enough of this smart nutrient is essential to prevent damage. Combining phospholipids with DHA, the omega-3 fat that helps to build the brain, may be particularily helpful. In animal studies giving extra DHA, the omega-3 fat, together with choline and uridine (a phospholipid precursor that our body makes), helps regenerate the brain's synapses, degeneration of which is thought to be a major cause of memory loss in Alzheimer's.[116] A pilot trial (details of which are on page 115) reported improvements in memory function in Alzheimer's patients given phospholipids providing 400mg of choline together with essential fats, antioxidants and homocysteine-lowering B vitamins.

One study conducted by researchers in Mexico found that giving choline to those with mild to moderate Alzheimer's improved memory over 6 months, while memory declined in those on the placebo.[117]

And some studies in which phosphatidyl choline has been given to people with no cognitive decline have shown clearly beneficial effects.[118] One placebo-controlled Californian trial involving 80 college students given a single 25g dose of phosphatidyl choline found a significant improvement in memory 90 minutes later.[119] By the way, there's a side benefit too – choline improves liver function.[120] I suspect that ensuring you are getting enough phosphatidyl choline is one of the best things you can do for your brain, and will produce memory improvements in those who are deficient.

But beyond that, I feel that taking PC is unlikely to constitute a miracle cure in people who already have Alzheimer's or other forms of dementia: to date, giving phosphatidyl choline to probable Alzheimer's patients has failed to result in improved memory. Studies focusing on people with vascular dementia (see page 33) have been more promising. A recent review of trials of those with vascular dementia concludes: 'In general, treatment with choline induced favourable effects on cognitive function in dementia disorders of vascular origin. These positive results should be regarded with caution due to the small number of patients included in controlled clinical trials.'[121]

DMAE – Stimulating the brain

It is much easier to get DMAE from the blood into the brain than to try to do that with phosphatidyl choline (which, if you'll remember, is synthesised from DMAE). So a number of researchers have tested the effects of DMAE on the brain. A chemical variant of DMAE has been marketed as the drug Deaner or Deanol, which has proven highly effective in numerous double-blind trials in helping those with learning, memory or behaviour problems, and attention deficit disorder. DMAE has been shown to reduce anxiety, stop the mind racing, improve concentration and promote learning.

The ability of DMAE to tune up your brain was well demonstrated in a 1996 German study with a group of adults who had cognitive problems.[122] The EEG brain waves of the participants were measured, and they were then given either placebos or DMAE. There were no changes in EEG for those on the placebos, but those taking DMAE showed improvements in brain wave patterns in parts of the brain that play an important role in memory, attention and flexibility of thinking.

This research was recently followed by a study in which 80 volunteers got to watch 'emotional' films. Some were given DMAE and others were given placebos. Both their brain wave patterns and their subjective feelings were monitored. In the words of the researchers, 'DMAE can be interpreted to induce a psychophysiological state of better feeling of well-being on both levels of analysis-mood and electrical pattern of brain activity in subjects suffering from borderline emotional disturbance.' So, not only do people report feeling better, their brain activity becomes healthier.

Here are some reports from people supplementing DMAE:

> I've been taking DMAE for several weeks and I've noticed an amazing difference in mood and concentration level.
> *AFB, Austin, Texas*

> I am currently taking 100mg of DMAE per day and notice a real difference in my alertness, energy level and decreased need for sleep.
> *RS, Seattle, Washington*

> I've been using DMAE with pantothenic acid and a good multivitamin for two months now. One of the first things I noticed was that I fall asleep faster and wake up with a clearer mind. I experience a much sounder, more restful sleep. I constantly feel more attuned to my creative potential and I'm always in a good mood. I truly feel alive and awake.
>
> *PW*[123]

These findings are impressive. But what about alleviating Alzheimer's? Does DMAE deliver a result for those with worsening memory? While animal studies have shown positive results,[124] to date there have been no impressive reversals in memory decline in people with Alzheimer's, although one study found improvement in mood, and a lessening of anxiety and irritability.[125]

If you take too much DMAE – that is, above 1500mg a day – it may even make things worse. One possible reason for this is that it can block the receptors for acetylcholine. I take 400mg a day and find it helps keep my mind and mood sharp and stable. Although the evidence in relation to Alzheimer's prevention is not there yet, there's good reason to add 100 to 500mg to your daily supplement regime. There is certainly no evidence of any downside at these kinds of daily doses. DMAE is found in a number of brain food formulas available in health food shops.

PS: Don't forget the phosphatidyl serine

While the jury is still out on DMAE's effect in people with dementia, the findings on phosphatidyl serine (PS), the second most abundant phospholipid in the brain, are encouraging regardless of the degree of memory impairment. In one study, supplementing PS improved the participants' memories to the level of people

12 years younger. Dr Thomas Crook from the Memory Assessment Clinic in Bethesda, Maryland, in the US, gave 149 people with age-associated memory impairment a daily dose of 300mg of PS or a placebo. When tested after 12 weeks, the ability of those taking PS to match names to faces (a recognised measure of memory and mental function) had vastly improved.[126]

More than 35 human studies spanning three decades, together with numerous animal studies, all indicate how important PS is for brain function. In animals with age-related memory decline it has proven highly beneficial.[127] Some 16 clinical trials indicate that PS benefits measurable cognitive functions which tend to decline with age, such as memory, learning, vocabulary skills and concentration, as well as mood, alertness and sociability. Studies have found that PS supplementation can also benefit those with only mild memory impairment,[128] and in addition to improving memory, can alleviate depressive symptoms and seasonal affective disorder (SAD).[129–30]

The secret of the memory-boosting properties of PS is probably its ability to help brain cells communicate, as it is a vital part of the structure of their receptor sites.

While the body can make its own PS, we rely on receiving some directly from diet – so it can be viewed as a semi-essential nutrient. The trouble is that modern diets are deficient in PS unless you happen to eat a lot of organ meats, in which case you may take in 50mg a day. A vegetarian diet, however, is unlikely to achieve even 10mg a day. Supplementing 100 to 300mg a day can make a real difference.

Eat your phospholipids

As we've seen in this chapter, the body can make phospholipids, but getting extra from your diet is even better. That means overcoming egg phobia, if you've developed it.

You may recall from Chapter 6 that egg yolk is a top source of phospholipids, and that eggs hardly deserve the 'unhealthy' label that was pinned on them some time ago. Yes, they're high in fat and cholesterol, but remember: the fat in that egg depends on what you feed the chicken. So if you feed it a diet rich in omega-3 fats, for example flax seeds or fishmeal, you get an egg high in omega-3s. Poached or boiled (but not fried) free-range organic eggs are a fantastic brain food, and the richest dietary source of choline.

And don't forget that cholesterol is essential for good health – it's used to make the sex hormones oestrogen, progesterone and testosterone, and the brain itself is cholesterol-rich. Eating eggs does not give you heart disease, and here's one of many studies that prove it: Dr Alfin-Slater of the University of California gave 25 healthy people with normal blood cholesterol levels two eggs per day (in addition to the other cholesterol-rich foods they were already eating as part of their normal diet) for eight weeks. A further 25 healthy people were given one extra egg per day for four weeks, then two extra eggs per day for the next four weeks. The results showed no change in blood cholesterol.[131] Other studies show the same thing.

In short, eggs are a superfood. So don't be shy – dig out the poaching pan and resurrect the breakfasts of your youth (and add hardboiled eggs to salads, sandwiches, curries and the like). Be aware, too, of other rich sources of choline: fish, liver, soya, peanuts, whole grains, nuts, pulses, citrus fruit, wheat germ and brewer's yeast.

Lecithin – a direct source

Lecithin is the best source of phospholipids, and widely available in health food shops, either as lecithin granules or capsules. As I indicated in Part 1, the ideal daily intake is 5g of lecithin, or half this if you take 'high PC' (phosphatidyl choline) lecithin. It's easy to include in your daily regime: add a tablespoon of lecithin, or a heaped teaspoon of high-PC lecithin, to your cereal in the morning, or take lecithin supplements. Most capsules provide 1200mg, so you would need four a day.

So, while an optimal intake of phospholipids helps your brain sing by improving the insulation around nerves, choline and serine are also brain nutrients in their own right.

Summary: getting enough phospholipids

- Add a tablespoon of lecithin granules, or a heaped teaspoon of high-PC lecithin, to your cereal every day.
- Or eat an egg a day, or six eggs a week – preferable free-range, organic and high in omega-3s.
- Supplement a brain food formula providing phosphatidyl choline, phosphatidyl serine and DMAE.

12

Alcohol – Why Moderation Works Best

FROM 'GETTING A BUZZ ON' to out-and-out bingeing, our love affair with alcohol doesn't seem to diminish. Far from it, in fact. The mad pace of our working lives is partly responsible, but the other pull comes from alcohol's seductive effect on our brain. The question – which we'll explore in this chapter – is, how safe is that effect over time?

It's certainly dramatic. Within minutes of consuming alcohol you start to loosen up, lower your inhibitions, and find yourself becoming more cheery and gregarious. This transformation is down to the release of dopamine, which stimulates you, followed by endorphins, which make you feel high, and then GABA, which makes you relax. The alcohol also gives your blood sugar a kick. Sounds good, doesn't it? It feels good too, and that's why we do it. This pleasant effect usually lasts for an hour or so.

Several drinks later, though, you might notice you're feeling irritable, depressed or even hostile (or others will). Your thinking and memory may get fuzzy. You could end up unsure of where you are, who you're with, and why you're there. You might then get sleepy or, on a bad night, pass out.

The relaxant effect of alcohol, which is so attractive after a hard day living off stress, stimulants and adrenalin, happens once the amount of alcohol ingested exceeds the ability of the liver to detoxify – and this happens very quickly. Needless to say, once you really start feeling the effects, mental alertness and intellectual performance take a downturn. In answer to the question about how safe this is – it all depends on how much you're drinking. If you're prone to bingeing or real blow-outs, you're doing yourself, and your brain, no favours. But as for the rest of us, how much is too much?

It's not smart to drink too much

Those who consume high levels of alcohol have lowered intellectual performance on testing, hardly surprisingly. But the same results have not been shown for moderate drinkers. In fact, one study by the National Institute for Public Health in the Netherlands found less risk of poor cognitive function among those who had one or two drinks a day, compared to abstainers.

While it is well known that excessive alcohol can lead to dementia, this is not the same thing as Alzheimer's disease. Researchers at the University of Pittsburgh psychiatry department in Pennsylvania compared the performance of alcoholics with dementia versus non-alcoholics with dementia. They found a very different pattern of poor mental function, suggesting that alcohol per se wasn't causing the same kind of brain damage as seen in Alzheimer's.[132]

This finding has been further confirmed by a recent study in which older people, from teetotallers to heavy drinkers, were given MRI scans to see whether there was a link between Alzheimer's-like damage in the brain and drinking. The researchers, from Rotterdam's Erasmus Medical Centre, took MRI scans of 1,074 people, aged 60 to 90, who did not have dementia. They were categorised according to their alcohol consumption from abstainers to very light (1 drink/week), light (1 drink/week to <1 drink/day), moderate (1 drink/day to <4 drinks/day), to heavy (4 drinks/day) drinkers. The team looked for damage or evidence of stroke,[133] and also measured hippocampus size, which is a strong indicator of Alzheimer's.

They found that the people with the healthiest brains – meaning the least damage, the least evidence of strokes and the least hippocampal shrinking – were not the very light drinkers or abstainers, but the light or moderate drinkers. Although the heavy drinkers came out worse, this finding suggests that while large amounts of alcohol damage the brain, a glass or two of wine a day does not, and may even reduce your risk of a stroke.

The evidence that a small amount of alcohol may even be brain-protective isn't based on one study alone. Studies in France have consistently shown that light to moderate alcohol drinkers have a lower incidence of both dementia and strokes, while heavy drinkers increase their risk of both diseases. So a moderate amount of what you fancy does you good.

How your liver protects your brain

The question is why? You can ask this question in two ways: why does excessive alcohol damage the brain, and why does moderate consumption appear to protect it? One piece of evidence comes from looking at liver function. While investigating the reason for memory and concentration problems in alcoholics, a team studying 280 patients with liver damage at the Johns Hopkins University School of Medicine in Baltimore, Maryland, found that their cognitive impairment was the result of liver damage rather than alcohol intake directly, as those with non-alcohol related liver damage had similar reductions in cognitive function.[134] This means that too much alcohol damages the liver; and since the liver 'detoxifies' the blood entering the brain, this in turn is bad news for your grey matter.

The liver detoxifies alcohol via the liver enzyme alcohol dehydrogenase. These enzymatic pathways depend on a good supply of antioxidant nutrients, especially vitamin C. But when alcohol intake impedes this preferred enzymatic pathway, the liver instead will metabolise alcohol to acetaldehyde. This very acidic and toxic metabolite creates an excess of what are called ketoacids in the blood, which cause hangovers – headache, nausea, mental and physical tiredness and aching muscles.

Yet even before alcohol gets to the liver it has negative effects in the gut, where it acts as an irritant. This increases the risk of intestinal permeability or a 'leaky gut', which in turn increases the risk of allergic reactions to absorbed particles of incompletely digested food, and to the ingredients within the alcoholic drink itself. For this reason, many beer and wine drinkers become allergic to yeast. About one in five people, on testing, have this sensitivity.

Wine drinkers may also become sensitive to sulphites, added to grapes to control their fermentation. Sulphites are also found in exhaust fumes, and the liver enzyme that detoxifies sulphites is dependent on molybdenum, a commonly deficient trace element. Better are organic, sulphite-free wines and champagne, the latter of which has the added bonus of being yeast-free.

Alcohol and homocysteine

But this doesn't answer why small amounts of alcohol seem to protect the brain. Let's take a look at homocysteine and alcohol. On the one hand, too much alcohol raises this important risk factor for Alzheimer's disease. In one study, for example, 60 normal, well-nourished people were given 30g of alcohol a day – the equivalent of 1.5 pints of beer, three regular glasses of wine, or three measures of spirits. At the end of the six weeks, whatever form of alcohol they'd been drinking, their homocysteine score was higher.[135]

But not all studies agree. A team led by researchers at the TNO Nutrition and Food Research Institute in the Netherlands decided to focus solely on beer and red wine. They gave volunteers either wine or beer to drink – an average of four glasses a night (the equivalent of 40g of alcohol) for 12 weeks. At the end of this time, while the homocysteine scores had gone up on red wine, they'd actually gone down on beer.[136]

And this team is not the only one to find that beer lowers homocysteine. A recent study from Pilsen in the Czech Republic gave over 500 volunteers a free litre of beer a day. (They had no problem getting recruits!) Once again, they found that this amount of beer was associated with slightly lower H scores, and higher folate and B12 levels in their bloodstreams.[137] Why? They speculated that the B vitamins in beer might have had a protective effect.

But before you rush out to your local pub for a few pints, be aware that a UK study comparing the effects of beer, wine and spirits in different amounts on the homocysteine levels of 350 obese people did not come up with the same finding. This team discovered that people consuming the equivalent of a drink a day had slightly lower H scores than those who abstained, and had slightly higher folate levels – but beer came out badly, while red wine came out on top. The people drinking red wine had an average score of 7.8; the white wine consumers scored 8.8; the beer and spirit drinkers, 9; and the abstainers, 9.4.[138] The study concluded that drinking around 100g of alcohol from red wine a week, which you'd get from a glass of wine a day, may slightly lower your H score.

Confused? It's hardly surprising if you are. But science is

sometimes like this! No doubt the beer and wine war will continue, with Dutch and French researchers battling for the best result for their national tipple. Either way, at this point it seems safe to say that light consumption of wine or beer won't hurt the brain and may even be protective, provided your liver is working fine and you are getting enough antioxidants, vitamin C and B vitamins. Exactly why moderate alcohol might be protective is not yet proven.

Alcohol and stress

Another possible explanation for the benefit of light to moderate alcohol consumption is that it reduces your stress levels and, as you'll see in Chapter 14, prolonged stress really does damage your brain. There is evidence for this alcoholic boost. Some researchers have found, for example, that light drinkers who are under stress suffer less from depression than abstainers and heavy drinkers under stress. So for some people, in some cases, a small amount of alcohol can help ease the stress of daily living.

On a more subtle level, according to psychologist Oscar Ichazo, alcohol is a great depleter of vital energy. In fact, he puts it top of the list, followed by heroin, tobacco, cocaine, barbiturates, anti-depressants, amphetamines, marijuana and caffeine. So, as a relaxant to combat excessive stress it has benefits, but with a considerable cost to overall energy. Of course, it's better not to be so stressed to start with.

How much is too much?

If you've weighed up the pros on alcohol and are about to buy a bottle to celebrate, I still recommend a word of caution. Alcohol does increase the risk of other diseases, most notably breast cancer.

A report in the journal *Cancer* found that among women who had a mother or sister with breast cancer, those who drank daily had almost 2.5 times the risk of breast cancer than those who did not drink alcohol at all. Another study reported that women whose diets were lowest in folate faced no greater cancer risk than women with higher-folate diets – if they were nondrinkers. But if they drank more than two alcoholic drinks a week, their breast cancer risk increased almost 60 per cent! The *Journal of the American Medical Association* (JAMA) earlier reported similar findings from a large-scale survey of female nurses.

How can you make sense of all these studies? Well, one clear suggestion is that getting enough of the homocysteine-lowering B vitamins is good news. Possibly, for those who are deficient, the amount provided in a beer or a glass of wine could be slightly beneficial and offset alcohol's negative effects. Also, having an optimal intake from diet and supplements may render alcohol less toxic.

However, it's a fine line, and moderation is the key word. I therefore recommend you drink no more than four glasses of red wine or beer a week, provided your homocysteine score is below 9. However, if you have a high H score, I recommend you avoid it completely until you are, at least, down to this level.

Summary: keeping alcohol intake safe

- Drink infrequently, ideally wine or beer, if your homocysteine score is above 9.
- Otherwise, have four alcoholic drinks a week.
- Keep following my suggestions for lowering homocysteine levels in Chapter 7, to make your consumption of alcohol doubly safe.

13

How Sugar Ages Your Brain

SUGAR, LIKE PETROL, is dangerous stuff. It's the fuel your brain runs off (that's why you can't think straight when you haven't eaten for hours), and all is well if it's used carefully. But if it is taken to excess, it can literally burn your brain – and the evidence shows that this is exactly what happens in many people who develop Alzheimer's. So in this chapter we'll be looking at how to keep that damage to a minimum by curbing our consumption of the white stuff.

Excessive amounts of sugar damage the brain because it forms toxic compounds called 'advanced glycation end products', or AGEs. Think of glucose, or blood sugar, as high-octane fuel. The goal of good nutrition is to deliver 'slow-releasing' carbohydrates that gradually break down into pure glucose fuel, which seeps into the bloodstream and is then escorted into cells, such as neurons, to help keep your energy high.

The hormone insulin is this escort, either ensuring hungry cells get their due, or dumping excess glucose into storage. It's a careful balancing act, and one that's likely to go wrong if you keep eating sugary or refined carbohydrates. The more you eat these, the more often you'll have peaks in your blood sugar levels, followed by troughs. And this seesawing will leave you tired and unable to concentrate, eventually experiencing 'blank-mind' episodes and fading memory.

If you continue to try to kickstart your system with sugar, resulting in more and more peaks and troughs, your body will become less and less responsive to its own insulin – and develop 'insulin resistance'. Someone in the grip of insulin resistance will produce more insulin in an attempt to get a response, a condition known as hyperinsulinemia, and get rebound blood sugar lows (hypoglycemia). Eventually, they will become so insulin resistant their blood sugar levels don't go down as they should. Type 2 diabetes is the result.

The bitter truth about sugar

So, what's all this got to do with preventing Alzheimer's? The answer is everything. Being insulin resistant or diabetic, having hyperinsulinema or hypoglycemia, have all been shown to tremendously increase a person's risk of developing Alzheimer's or dementia.

There are probably many reasons why an upset in blood sugar control damages the brain, but one that stands out is the fact that occasional blood sugar peaks actually sugar-coat proteins, and damage them, creating damaging AGEs. A lifetime of sugar abuse, glycation (adverse interactions between glucose and proteins, for instance) and AGE creation lead to more and more artery and brain damage. The more the arteries become damaged, the worse the circulation to the brain and the less reliable the supply of nutrients, including glucose, becomes. So, ironically, eating too much sugar can lead to temporary glucose starvation to cells, as well as damage caused by excess glycation.

AGEs are not only bad for the brain – they also damage your skin, producing wrinkles and age spots. These damaged proteins produce 50 times the number of free radicals that non-glycated proteins do, and promote inflammation in the brain as well as the skin, joints and other organs.

So oxidants and AGEs constitute a double whammy for your brain. Researchers now believe that AGEs may be a player in Alzheimer's disease because they have been found in the neurofibrillary tangles that characterise the condition, and the formation of beta-amyloid plaque is significantly accelerated by the presence of AGEs.

The glucose/Alzheimer's link

There has been much research into the links between blood sugar and Alzheimer's. For example, researchers at Columbia University in New York studied 683 people without dementia who were 65 years or older for five and a half years. During that time, twice as many of the participants with high insulin levels developed dementia when compared to those with normal insulin levels. Also, the people with high insulin levels had the greatest decline in memory.[139] An Italian study of people free of dementia and diabetes showed that high insulin levels were strongly associated with poorer mental function.[140]

Meanwhile, a six-year Swedish study of 1,301 people aged 75 and over showed that those with diabetes were one and a half times more likely to develop dementia. The risk was even greater in diabetics who also had high blood pressure or heart disease.[141] A number of other studies have also shown a strong association between diabetes and cognitive decline.[142–4]

One of the best measures of your blood sugar control is something called *glycosylated haemoglobin.* You can buy home test kits that measure your level. It actually measures how sugar coated your red blood cells are. You want to have a score below 5.5 per cent. Researchers at the University of California, San Francisco, studied 1,983 postmenopausal women and found those with glycosylated haemoglobin levels of 7 per cent or higher were four times more likely to develop mild cognitive impairment or dementia than those with levels lower than 7 per cent.[145]

Why sugar is addictive

It's one thing to know that sugar is bad for your brain, but another to quit eating it – especially when the desire for something sweet is one of the body's strongest instincts. Your body and brain are much more responsive to deficiency than to having too much. There's a simple reason for this. In evolutionary terms, starvation is a much more likely, and threatening, situation than today's danger of excess. Consequently, we are all programmed to love sugar, which with its high-energy kick offers a fast way out of any potential starvation.

The way this programming works is that sugar causes the release of dopamine and beta-endorphin, two neurotransmitters that make you feel good. Heroin and morphine also evoke a beta-endorphin response, while cocaine evokes a dopamine response. So the more you have, the more you want, as you become less and less responsive to it. In short, you'd become addicted to it[146–50] and no addiction is easy to break.

The late Dr Emanuel Cheraskin (Professor of Medicine and Dentistry, University of Alabama) calls sugar 'the mother of all addiction'.[151] Dr Candace Pert, Research Professor in the Department of Physiology and Biophysics at Georgetown University Medical Center in Washington DC, says, 'I consider sugar to be a drug, a highly purified plant product that can become addictive. Relying on an artificial form of glucose – sugar – to give us a quick pick-me-up is analogous to, if not as dangerous as, shooting up heroin.'[152] Pert is one of the chief scientists involved in the discovery of the central role endorphins play in addiction.

I'll explain more about how to cut back on sugar, and what to eat instead, in Part 3, but for now, I'd like to tell you about another reason too many of us indulge in it.

If you are feeling depressed, especially in winter, there's a good chance your brain levels of serotonin are low. Serotonin is made from a constituent of protein, the amino acid tryptophan. However, ironically, eating a meal containing tryptophan doesn't raise brain levels of tryptophan as high as eating a carbohydrate meal does. This anomaly was discovered by Professor Richard Wurtman in a series of studies at Massachusetts Institute of Technology. He fed people standard American high-protein breakfasts versus high-carbohydrate breakfasts and found that only the latter boosted serotonin levels, despite containing no tryptophan![153] The reason for this anomaly is that tryptophan in the bloodstream competes very badly with all the other amino acids in protein, so little gets across into the brain. However, when you eat a carbohydrate food such as a banana, this causes insulin to be released into the bloodstream – and insulin carries tryptophan into the brain.

This may be why depressed people instinctly crave sweet foods to give them a lift. They cause a surge of insulin, which carries tryptophan into the brain, causing serotonin levels to rise! So, if you find sugar improves your mood no end, you are probably low in serotonin.

The trouble is, eating sweet, carbohydrate-rich foods isn't a very good way of getting happy. Most carbohydrate snacks are high in refined sugar and fat, and also make you fat, which is depressing in itself. The solution is to supplement a tryptophan-rich food, such as turkey, with a healthy carbohydrate snack such as an apple. This combination is much more effective in raising the brain's level of serotonin, which will not only improve your mood, but also reduce your appetite, especially for sugary foods. That's why tryptophan can also help you lose weight.

Summary: saying no to sugar and going for slow-release carbs

- Eat wholefoods – whole grains, lentils, beans, nuts, seeds, fresh fruit and vegetables – and avoid refined, white and overcooked foods.
- Eat five servings a day of dark green, leafy and root vegetables such as watercress, carrots, sweet potatoes, broccoli, Brussels sprouts, spinach, green beans or peppers, either raw or lightly cooked.
- Eat three or more servings a day of fresh fruit, preferably apples, pears and/or berries.
- Eat four or more servings a day of whole grains such as rice, rye, oats, wholewheat, corn, quinoa as cereal, breads, pasta or pulses.
- Avoid any form of sugar or added sugar.
- Dilute fruit juices and only eat dried fruit infrequently in small quantities, preferably soaked or with a small handful of nuts or seeds.

14

The Cortisol Connection – Why Stress Makes You Stupid

STRESS HAS AN ENORMOUS impact on your memory and your risk of developing Alzheimer's. And this isn't just some vague, generalised effect: it is very specific indeed. All animals are geared up to produce the adrenal hormones adrenalin and cortisol when under stress. These switch on during the 'fight/flight' reaction, which gears you up fast for action. The effect of these hormones is quite remarkable, instantly raising your blood sugar levels, and pumping fuel into muscles for an instant response. Everything else stops – digestion, normal bodily repair, your immune system all grind to a halt. A simple example of this is a dry mouth, which you might experience when you're asked to make a presentation. It's a sign that the stress reaction is shutting down digestion, starting with the production of saliva.

The immediate effect of stress on memory is to improve it. This is why you can remember all the tiny details in that car smash you had. It's all part of our programming, because at threatening times you have to remember everything and act quickly.

But extreme stress like this is rare, and over quickly. The problem is that nowadays many of us are in a permanent state of stress, for reasons largely generated in our heads rather than as a result of actual physical danger. Psychological stress, be it the need to perform at work, relationship problems, or just general anxiety about life, causes a non-stop output of cortisol, and research is showing that this is a very bad thing for the brain.

In this chapter we'll look at how to wean ourselves off this kind of damaging 'background' stress, thus lowering our cortisol levels. But first, check yourself out on the Stress Check below.

Stress Check

Score 1 for each 'yes' answer.

	Yes	No
Do you have difficulty relaxing?	☐	☐
Do you often find yourself feeling irritable?	☐	☐
Do you worry about little events of the day, and find you are unable to shut your mind off?	☐	☐
Do you smoke or drink excessively (especially by others' standards)?	☐	☐
Are you somewhat addicted to caffeinated drinks?	☐	☐
Are you competitive and aggressive in the things you do?	☐	☐
Do you find it hard to relate to people?	☐	☐
Do you find you are impatient with others?	☐	☐
Do you eat quickly?	☐	☐

Do you take on too much?	☐	☐
Do you have difficulty delegating?	☐	☐
Do you have aching limbs or recurrent headaches?	☐	☐
Do you have a dry mouth and sweaty palms?	☐	☐
Do you feel a lack of interest in sex?	☐	☐
Are your muscles tense?	☐	☐
Do you have problems sleeping?	☐	☐

If your score is:

Below 5: You're in fine shape, able to take life in your stride.

5 to 10: You are quite stressed; pay attention to these warning signs. This is the only body you have: treat it well. You'll see how to do this in the following pages.

More than 10: You are very stressed and it is probably having a negative effect on your brain.

How cortisol damages your brain

According to Professor Robert Sapolsky, one of America's top stress experts from Stanford University in California, cortisol damages your brain. Raised levels of cortisol have been linked to poorer memory and a shrinking of the brain's memory sorting centre. Short-term stress leaves the neurons in the hippocampus, that key area linked to the origin of Alzheimer's, a bit shaken up. What this means is that they are less likely to recover from, say, a high level of oxidants, or raised homocysteine. Cortisol also makes the toxic protein beta-amyloid more toxic.

In animals, the effects of stress on the brain are undeniable.

After only two weeks of raised cortisol levels, the dendrites – the 'arms' of brain cells that reach out to connect with other brain cells – start to shrivel up, according to research carried out by Sapolsky.[154] But there's good news: the damage isn't permanent. Stop the stress and the dendrites grow back.

What happens to us humans, however? Does our brain bounce back from stress? Three different types of study shed light on this vital question, and the news isn't good. The first involves people with a rare disease called Cushing's syndrome, caused by a tumour of the adrenal or pituitary glands. People with this condition make too much cortisol, and they are prone to atrophy of the hippocampus, and dementia. However, when the tumour is removed and the cortisol levels drop back to normal, the brain repairs the damage. This means the neurons weren't actually dead, just disabled.

Studies of people with post-traumatic stress disorder reveal a darker picture. Using a brain imaging technique, Douglas Bremner of Yale University in the US has shown that the part of the brain responsible for learning and memory is smaller in patients with post-traumatic stress disorder, and that this correlates with poorer memory.[155] What these studies also show is irreversible atrophy of the hippocampus. There's no recovery.

Depression and anxiety

So, who is permanently stressed? There's a good chance that people who suffer from depression are living in a state of anxiety. Recent research has shown that about 15 per cent of depressed people have highly elevated cortisol levels, atrophy of the hippocampus and, 15 years later, show no sign of recovery! This is extremely bad news, especially when you know it's backed up by many studies showing that cortisol levels are significantly higher in Alzheimer's patients than in controls, and that the higher the cortisol, the worse the symptoms.[156–8]

None of this is normal ageing. In fact, research at McGill University in Canada followed up a group of 70–year-olds for five years. Only those with high cortisol levels were found to have shrunken hippocampuses and worsening memory.

Reacting stressfully to life's twists and turns isn't the only way to raise your cortisol levels. Another way is to take a steroid drug such as prednisolene. In the US there are 60 million prescriptions for steroid drugs each year, and an estimated 30 million in England. The concern is not so much about that steroid cream you use when your eczema flares up, but about the long-term use of steroid drugs such as painkillers and anti-inflammatories.

The moral of this story is 'don't react stressfully'. Of course, that's easier to say than to do. Life is maniacally speeded-up for most people in the 21st century, there is less job security, and too many of us are constantly striving to achieve some imaginary goal, like mice chasing elusive cheese. It's key to reappraise your goals and your priorities so there's more fun and balance in your life, and less endless overload. Don't underestimate the effects of non-stop stress and anxiety. Reacting in this way can become habit-forming. Find a way to break the habit and give your brain time to recover.

Summary: lowering stress and cortisol levels

- If something riles you, express it. Depression is often anger without enthusiasm. It's much better to let it out – as long as you do it responsibly and appropriately.
- Go for a run, beat up a cushion, or buy a punch bag. Physical release of stress immediately lowers cortisol.
- Get used to it. People in high-stress jobs do often adapt. If you become used to high stress, then lower your stress level, cortisol levels often drop accordingly.

- Stay in control. We often react stressfully when we perceive ourselves to be out of control. So learn how to manage your life and your time so you do have a sense of control. Before you take on a new project, finish an old one. Unfinished business is a major source of stress.
- Talk to someone. For us humans, in fact all primates, social connectedness is one of the most predictive indicators of health. We need people to talk to, shoulders to cry on. Don't isolate yourself. Make new friends. People with depression experience relief even by keeping a diary. Self-reflection seems to help.
- Learn how to meditate, take up yoga or start practising t'ai chi. These are great ways of de-stressing, and they're discussed in more detail in Chapter 19.

15

Give Your Brain a Heavy Metal Detox

SOME MINERALS ARE KEY to health; others are highly toxic if they enter our bodies. Minerals are elements, and each has special properties. The essential elements, such as zinc, are needed to drive enzymes and chemical reactions in the brain and body. Toxic elements, on the other hand, interfere with that process and may play a role in worsening memory. And even essential elements become toxic in excess: a good example is copper.

Overall, most people accumulate undesirable elements such as aluminium, mercury, lead, copper and cadmium throughout life, while simultaneously becoming increasingly deficient in essential ones, such as magnesium, zinc, chromium, manganese and selenium. Keeping your levels of toxic elements low is a wise precaution, and in this chapter we'll be looking in detail at how to do that.

Aluminium – trouble in store

A mass of studies show an increased accumulation of aluminium in the plaques of Alzheimer's sufferers. What isn't clear is whether this is a cause or a consequence of the disease. However, there are good reasons to suspect aluminium could be a factor in memory loss.

First, there's no question that aluminium, in excess, does lead to the development of the neurofibrillary tangles. This has been shown in animal studies. Secondly, aluminium has been found to be high in the plaques and tangles in the brains of those who died from Alzheimer's. Thirdly, a number of surveys have found higher rates of dementia in areas where the aluminium levels in the environment, most notably the water supply, are high. Lastly, giving an aluminium 'chelator' desferroximine, which helps to take aluminium out of the brain, has been shown to slow the progression of Alzheimer's disease.[159]

Researchers at the University of Torino in Italy studied 64 former foundry workers who had been exposed to aluminium dust. They found much higher levels of aluminium in the blood of these people compared with people of similar age who had not been exposed. In memory tests, the ex-foundry workers with the highest levels of aluminium performed the worst.[160]

In a study in the 1980s of 647 Canadian gold miners who had routinely inhaled aluminium since the 1940s (this used to be a common practice, thought to prevent silica poisoning), all tested in the 'impaired' range for cognitive function, suggesting a clear link between aluminium and memory loss.[161] Moreover, a number of recent reviews of the current scientific literature have kept aluminium firmly on the map of potential contributors to Alzheimer's.[162–3]

However, in another study, researchers at the University of Oxford didn't find aluminium in the brain tissue of people who died of Alzheimer's.[164] Along with another group of researchers from the National University of Singapore, they used a new technique for studying brain tissue called nuclear microscopy, which allows the examination of brain tissue without first 'staining' or 'fixing' it. Both groups of researchers believe that it is this staining and fixing process that causes the appearance of high levels of aluminium, because the staining and fixing chemicals themselves include aluminium.[165] But researchers at Queen's University in Ontario, Canada, who analysed brain tissue alongside the fixing and staining chemicals, concluded that the aluminium didn't come from the chemicals but had built up over the person's life.[166]

While there is plenty of evidence that aluminium has a damaging effect on the brain and may be a contributor to the development of Alzheimer's, it is not conclusive. Nevertheless, the toxic effect of aluminium on brain health cannot be ruled out either, and therefore I recommend that you limit your exposure to aluminium as far as possible.

This might seem daunting at first. Aluminium is all around us – in aspirin, antacids, antidiarrhoeal drugs, cake mixes, self-raising flour, processed cheese, baking powder, drinking water, milk, talcum powder, tobacco smoke, drink cans, cooking utensils and pans, air pollution compounds and aluminium foil. Yet it is poorly absorbed into the body unless you are zinc deficient – and the problem is that most people are. Aluminium also becomes much more absorbable in acidic conditions. So if, for example, you boil tea containing tannic acid, or rhubarb, which contains oxalic acid, in an old aluminium pan, you can leach aluminium from the pan into the food or drink.

It's important to identify the potential sources in your diet and environment and reduce or eliminate them. I have often seen high levels in those who grill food directly on aluminium foil, for example.

Your aluminium level is easily tested in a hair mineral analysis. There's more on this and how to reduce your level if it is high at the end of this chapter.

Mercury – why hatters were mad

Mercury has been a known brain toxin for centuries. The saying 'mad as a hatter' originated because mercury was used during hat manufacture in the 18th and 19th centuries. Over time, hatters began to have twitches and tremors, and eventually hallucinations culminating in madness – all the result of mercury exposure.

But is mercury a factor in Alzheimer's? And if so, where is it coming from, how do you test for it and what can you do about it if you are mercury-toxic?

Mercury is very toxic indeed and small amounts reach us from contaminated foods and from tooth fillings. So-called 'silver' or amalgam fillings are about 50 per cent mercury. Also of particular concern is fish caught in waters polluted with mercury. Mercury is used in a number of chemical processes, and accidents and illegal dumping have led to increased mercury levels in some areas, including the English Channel. There are also natural sources (see page 166). Larger fish like tuna, swordfish, marlin and shark have the highest levels of mercury because they eat smaller fish which also contain mercury, and it accumulates.

Mercury is also used as a constituent of thimerosal, a preservative found in many vaccines, including diphtheria, hepatitis, tetanus and flu. Currently, however, thimerosal is not added to MMR (although it had been until quite recently), Hib, polio, meningitis C or BCG vaccines used in the UK.

Researchers at the University of Kentucky in the US compared the brains of 10 people who had died with Alzheimer's with the brains of 10 people without memory problems who had died at similar ages. The biggest difference in mineral levels in the two sets of brains was that the Alzheimer's brains had high levels of mercury, especially in the areas of the brain that relate to memory.[167] At the University of Basel in Switzerland, researchers have found that blood levels of mercury in Alzheimer's patients are more than double those of people of similar age without Alzheimer's. The patients with early-onset Alzheimer's had the highest mercury levels of all.[168]

Trace amounts of mercury can cause the type of damage to the brain that is characteristic of Alzheimer's, according to research at the University of Calgary Faculty of Medicine in Canada – strongly suggesting that the small amounts we are exposed to, for example from amalgam fillings, may be contributing to memory loss. This fascinating piece of research showed that mercury causes degeneration in the brain cells and the formation of neurofibrillary tangles.[169–70] (The research team created a video of this experiment which you can view for free on the internet. Just type in the website address: http://commons.ucalgary.ca/mercury/.)

Some studies, however, suggest that increased levels of mercury are not a factor in Alzheimer's disease.[171–2] But we've seen how other research indicates that mercury may be present in greater amounts in the brains of some Alzheimer's sufferers, where it is quite possibly causing some damage. If so, where is it coming from?

A World Health Organization report from 1991 states that daily exposure to mercury from dental amalgams ranged from 3 to 17 micrograms per day, compared with up to 2.3 micrograms per day from fish and seafood and 0.3 micrograms per day from other food sources. We all consume, on average, 1mcg of mercury a day from food, water and air.

And those amalgam fillings could be leaching more mercury into the body than many suppose. The Calgary team has found that the more mercury you have in your mouth, the more you will have in your brain. The researchers placed radioactively labelled mercury (for ease of tracking) into the teeth of sheep and monkeys. Within 30 days of placing the fillings, substantial quantities of mercury appeared in the lung, gut, and jaw tissue, and ultimately became stored in other parts of the body such as the liver, kidney, brain, heart and glands. However, other studies fail to show any link between the number of mercury fillings, their size or length of time in the mouth, and brain levels of mercury.[173]

All fish contain mercury, and generally the larger the fish, the more mercury they contain, as we saw above. So, for example, the highest is shark (1.5mcg per kg), followed by swordfish (1.4), marlin (1.1) and tuna (0.4). Salmon and trout tend to be very low (around 0.05mcg). But contrary to popular opinion, most of this mercury isn't from man-made pollution. Humans have always been exposed to mercury from volcanoes, and there are plenty of those on the ocean bed.

In order to assess whether there were any effects on the brain caused by relatively low levels of mercury absorbed through eating fish, researchers at the University of Cagliari in Sardinia, Italy, compared 22 men who regularly ate tuna with relatively high mercury content, with 22 men who did not. The levels of mercury in the urine and blood of the fish-eaters was clearly linked with the quantity of fish eaten per week, and was four to 16 times higher than in the non-fish eaters. The mental agility of the fish-eaters was significantly worse in tests of reaction time and 'finger tapping speed'.[174]

On top of this, mercury seems to accumulate with age. This was demonstrated in a study of women aged 15 to 45 living in remote regions of the Amazon jungle, who ate fish twice per day. The study showed that 82 per cent of the women tested had mercury levels above the 'normal' range and the level of mercury in their bodies (measured by hair analysis) increased with age.[175]

Although the jury is still out on the links between mercury and Alzheimer's, it is certainly wise to reduce your exposure to this highly toxic metal. Beyond fish, fillings and vaccines, you are unlikely to be exposed to significant amounts of mercury in the environment, since its extreme toxicity means it has to be kept under very controlled conditions. But be aware that it may be present in some fungicides, insecticides, household products, cosmetics and medicines. It always pays to check labels.

At the end of this chapter I will tell you how to test for mercury levels and what to do if you find that your levels are high.

The copper controversy

Copper is both an essential mineral and a toxic contaminant. Copper deficiencies are rare, except in people with diets very high in refined foods, largely because much of the water we drink travels through copper pipes. These leach small amounts of copper into water. However, if you live in a soft-water area or in a house with new copper piping that hasn't yet got calcified, you can be exposed to higher levels of copper. The most recognised effects of copper on mental health are anxiety and paranoia, but can it affect your memory?

Dr Ashley Bush from Harvard Medical School, with colleagues from the University of Melbourne, Australia, have proposed that beta-amyloid is a 'metalloprotein' (meaning a combination of metals and protein) that contains zinc, copper and iron. They believe that beta-amyloid mops up surplus metals in the brain, causing it to build up and also produce more hydrogen peroxide, a toxic free radical that ages brain cells by oxidising them. Copper encourages this effect, while zinc appears to render beta-amyloid less harmful. This theory has only been put to the test in a small trial where clioquinol, a drug that prevents copper and zinc binding to beta-amyloid, was given to Alzheimer's patients. The drug reduced deterioration in these people's condition.[176] One survey found that those with both high copper intakes and high saturated fat intakes had faster memory decline with age, although copper intake alone was associated with better cognition.[177]

Zinc's beneficial effect on beta-amyloid is borne out by a theory put forward by Dr J. Constantinidis of the University of Geneva Medical School's Department of Psychiatry. Constantinidis blames zinc deficiency for allowing heavy metals to become problematic.[178] He reckons that beta-amyloid production disturbs the blood–brain barrier, allowing toxic metals to enter the brain, where they displace zinc in some enzymes and disturb brain metabolism. A greater concentration of zinc in the brain tissue may prevent this.

The beta-amyloid/copper connection has appeared in a number of other studies showing that copper is involved in its formation. However, as we saw earlier, the evidence isn't yet conclusive on whether these plaques are a cause or a consequence of Alzheimer's.

Aside from drinking water that has passed through copper piping, other causes of high copper levels include copper pots and pans, copper sulphate used as an algaecide in swimming pools, the contraceptive pill (oestrogen encourages copper build-up) and even copper IUDs and copper bracelets. Or it can be the result of a deficiency in vitamin C, B3 or zinc, as all of these are copper antagonists. Drinking filtered or bottled water will reduce your intake of copper from drinking water.

At the end of this chapter I tell you how to test for copper levels and what to do if you find that your levels are high.

Hair mineral analysis – your heavy-metal MOT

There's a simple way to find out if you have a build-up of heavy or toxic minerals: a hair mineral analysis. Analysing a small amount of hair provides an effective screen, not only for the bad guys such as aluminium, mercury and copper, but also for the good guys such as zinc, selenium, sulphur and so on. For around £50, it's well worth it. It's best to arrange your test through a clinical nutritionist or other suitably qualified health professional who can help you to interpret the results and advise what you need to do to remedy any excesses of the bad guys or deficiencies in the good guys. (See Resources on page 246 for details on how to find a clinical nutritionist and arrange a hair mineral analysis.)

There is one caveat regarding hair analysis, to do with mercury. Mercury is not as well represented in hair samples as the other minerals, for a number of reasons. The mercury can end up sequestered deep in body tissues, while still remaining sparse in your hair, for instance. But you can assume that if the test shows a significant amount of mercury, then you have at least that amount in your body.

There is, however, another test you can use specifically to test for mercury – the Kelmer Test. This involves drinking a solution containing a 'chelating agent' – a chemical that will bind to mercury and drag it out of your body cells – and then measuring the mercury in a urine sample. While this test is more accurate for mercury, the downside is that it stirs up the mercury in your body and may make you feel quite unwell. So it is not recommended for people who are not in robust health except under the direct supervision of a suitably qualified nutritionist or other health professional.

How to detoxify your brain

So, if you find that you have high levels of the bad guys, what should you do, besides reducing your exposure to them as outlined so far in this chapter?

Since your body is constantly striving to rid itself of all toxins, the first thing to do is support this process. First, that means focusing on your liver, the body's primary organ of detoxification. It's a very busy organ with over 600 functions, so to help it to work more efficiently, you need to reduce its overall workload. This means keeping your intake of all toxins to a minimum, including caffeine, alcohol, nicotine, artificial additives and preservatives and some unnecessary over-the-counter medications. You also need to feed it with plenty of nutrients, especially magnesium (found in leafy green vegetables), B vitamins (whole grains), and antioxidants (fresh fruit and vegetables).

You need to think about how toxins are excreted, too. Their

main route out of the body is via your bowel or kidneys. So you'll need plenty of fibre in your diet, enough to ensure regular bowel movements (two to three per day is ideal). Pectin – found in apples and beetroot – along with alginic acid from seaweed and non-starchy vegetables, are all great sources of fibre, as are psyllium seed husks, a fibre supplement. Drinking one to two litres of water a day is just as important, as this supports not just your bowel but also your kidneys and liver.

After a hair mineral analysis, or simply if you want to help your body detoxify further, you can do the following to reduce levels of specific metals:

- The most important nutrient for reducing aluminium levels is vitamin C. Vitamin C is found in highest quantities in fresh fruit (kiwi fruit is C-rich) and vegetables.
- Mercury removal is also helped by selenium, zinc, vitamin C and sulphur. Selenium is found in seeds, Brazil nuts and seafood; zinc is found in seeds, nuts, eggs and oysters; and vitamin C, as we've seen, stars in a number of fresh fruits and vegetables. For sulphur, look to garlic, onions and eggs.
- You may also like to consider having your mercury fillings removed. It is imperative that removal of mercury fillings is carried out by a dentist who specialises in this procedure. See Resources on page 246 for details of how to find a mercury-free dentist. Since the exposure to mercury is greatest during the placing and removal of mercury fillings, it is essential that the proper precautions are taken to protect you.
- For excess copper, increase your intake of zinc, vitamin C and vitamin B3 (niacin). Niacin is found in mushrooms, tuna and asparagus.

Summary: keeping heavy metals to a minimum

- Reduce your exposure to all sources of the toxic metals and limit your intake of swordfish, marlin and shark to no more than twice a month and tuna to no more than three times a month.
- Support overall detoxification by reducing your intake of all toxins – that is, avoid caffeine, alcohol, nicotine, sugar, artificial additives and preservatives.
- Improve the removal of toxins from your body by eating a high-fibre diet and drinking plenty of filtered or natural mineral water (at least one to two litres every day).
- Make sure you supplement at least 1g of vitamin C, 10mg of zinc and 50mcg of selenium every day.
- Have a hair mineral analysis (see Resources, page 249) and consult a clinical nutritionist who can advise you on specific supplements to help remove any excesses in toxic metals.

16

Herbs that Help Boost Memory

HERBAL MEDICINE IS OUR oldest form of 'chemical' medicine, and three herbs with a track record stretching back thousands of years are proving beneficial in keeping mind and memory sharp. This dynamic trio is ginkgo biloba, ginseng, and an extract from the periwinkle plant known as vinpocetine, and in this chapter we'll explore the properties of each in turn.

Ginkgo biloba – the circulation booster

Ginkgo biloba has been used by the Chinese for thousands of years, both as a memory booster and as an aphrodisiac. It's also one of the oldest known tree species on the planet. While studies on younger people haven't always proven its benefit, studies on older people, especially those with circulation problems, have shown encouraging results during the 1990s.

A review of the first 10 studies testing ginkgo's effects on people with circulation problems, carried out at the University of Limburg in the Netherlands, found significant improvement in memory, concentration, energy and mood.[179] Then, in 1997, a comprehensive double-blind placebo-controlled trial carried out in France found remarkable improvement in the speed of cognitive processing in 60 to 80–year-olds, almost comparable to those of healthy young people, when given 320mg or 600mg a day.[180] (Interestingly, the higher dose didn't work any better than the lower one.) A review of all studies to date, in 2002, concluded 'promising evidence of improvement in cognition and function with ginkgo.'[181]

This spawned tremendous medical interest in ginkgo in the context of dementia, and three further trials. The results, however, weren't so encouraging. Two failed to find a significant effect in people who had dementia,[182–3] while the third showed some improvement in elderly people who had not been diagnosed with dementia.[184] In this last study, 262 people aged 60 and older were given ginkgo at a dose of 160mg a day, or a placebo, for six weeks. Those on ginkgo had significantly improved memory function.

Ginkgo may therefore have a role to play in prevention, but does not seem to have a remarkable effect once a person actually has dementia. A recent review concludes that the results with ginkgo are 'inconsistent and unconvincing, but not dangerous, for dementia'.[185]

Ginkgo biloba may also be helpful in depression in the elderly – it has been shown to increase serotonin receptor sites in older but not in young rats, suggesting that it may block an age-related loss of serotonin receptors.[186]

Active ingredients and safety

Just because ginkgo is a plant, it doesn't mean it functions as a nutrient. Nutrients are essential biochemicals that we depend on.

There is no real evidence that ginkgo contains such compounds, although of course it does contain active compounds of its own. For this reason, it is very important to understand not only how a herb works, but also whether it has any undesirable side-effects.

Ginkgo contains two phytochemicals, ginkgo flavone glycoside and terpene lactone, which appear to be the main players in its healing effect. It appears to work by improving circulation in two ways. First, it makes your blood less sticky by reducing what's called platelet adhesion – platelets being tiny disks that form part of the blood. Aspirin has the same effect. Ginkgo's second healing mechanism is that it promotes nitric oxide, a molecule that keeps your veins and arteries dilated enough to ease blood flow. Viagra also works by promoting nitric oxide. (And like Viagra, ginkgo appears to enhance sexual performance – a pleasant side-effect of this memory-boosting herb. One trial[187] found that 84 per cent of people taking 240mg of ginkgo had enhanced desire, excitement and orgasm.

But there's more to ginkgo's action than just stimulating circulation. It also apparently increases the uptake of choline, and makes the brain more sensitive to the effects of both acetylcholine and serotonin. And it has a mild GABA-promoting effect, giving it mild relaxant properties.[188]

No serious side-effects have been reported in the now numerous trials testing ginkgo. There have been a few reports, however, of increased bleeding, almost always in people also taking a blood-thinning drug such as aspirin or warfarin. So there is a real need for caution in combining ginkgo with these drugs, and I do not recommend you do so without your doctor's consent. (Note that while vitamin E and omega-3s also have blood-thinning properties, the amounts I recommend in this book are compatible with taking ginkgo.) I have also known of a couple of reports of nosebleeds in people taking larger amounts of ginkgo. This is certainly an indication to lower the amount of ginkgo you take.

Since trials with ginkgo show that more is not necessarily

better, that daily intakes of between 160 and 320mg a day are effective, and that people seem to have different levels of sensitivity to it, my advice is to start with 40mg a day as a basic preventive dose, and increase to no more than 350mg a day.

As with all herbs, the amount you need depends on the potency of that particular source of ginkgo. The best way to gauge this is to look at its flavonoid concentration, which determines its strength. The better products state this. The recommended flavonoid concentration is 24 per cent, of which one would take 20 to 100mg up to three times a day. Ginkgo is sometimes also contained in brain food formulas.

Vinpocetine – power of the periwinkle

Much like the herb ginkgo biloba, vinpocetine also improves blood flow and circulation, thus helping to deliver oxygen to the brain. Vinpocetine is actually an extract from the periwinkle plant (*Vinca major*), a popular garden flower.

Research carried out at the University of Surrey in the UK gave 203 people with memory problems either a placebo or vinpocetine. This and other studies have shown that people taking vinpocetine experience a significant improvement in their cognitive performance.[189–90] Remarkably, improvements in concentration, memory recall and learning have been reported after just one dose. One double-blind crossover study showed a significant improvement in memory just an hour after taking 40mg of vinpocetine.[191]

The herb is recommended for those who've noticed a decline in their memory, concentration, learning speed, neuro-muscular coordination and reaction time, or impaired hearing or vision.

However, research shows that vinpocetine is particularly protective in cases where blood flow to the brain is diminished, usually by cerebral atherosclerosis (a condition in which a build-up of plaque clogs the arteries that supply oxygen to the brain), or during a mini-stroke. Like ginkgo, it may also help people with the ear condition tinnitus, which can be caused by such circulation problems.

The secrets of vinpocetine's success in enhancing mind and memory are many. Like ginkgo, vinpocetine inhibits platelet aggregation, thus stopping blood cells from clumping together and clogging the blood vessels. But studies also show that it widens blood vessels in the brain – thus boosting circulation and allowing red blood cells to more easily pass through narrow veins, improving oxygen delivery.

Brain cells not only need a constant, good supply of oxygen. They also need energy, and vinpocetine has been shown to enhance energy production in brain cells. By speeding up the transport of glucose and oxygen to the brain, as well as their use once they get there, vinpocetine may reduce the effects of both strokes and the less dramatic mini-strokes that can lead to dementia.

Finally, vinpocetine has been found to stimulate noradrenergic neurons in an area of the brain called the locus coeruleus. These neurons affect the function of the cerebral cortex – the part of the brain we use to think, plan and act. As we age, they decline in number, impairing concentration, alertness and the speed with which we process information.

While vinpocetine is less well researched than ginkgo, the trials to date are promising – there is no real indication of negative effects and plenty of positive ones.[192] You need about 10 to 40mg of vinpocetine a day for these positive effects.

Ginseng – tonic for the mind

Ginseng is one of the most widely used and researched energy-promoting herbs, and there's no doubt that it works in this context. The active ingredients are called ginsenosides. There are many different ones, each with specific effects. Most of the modern-day research on ginseng has been done on the clinical effects of single components.

Ginseng's effect on physical energy is one thing; but can it also boost mental acuity? In 1988, a German university professor, E. Ploss, published a summary and analysis of studies on the clinical use of Asian ginseng, which was followed in 1990 by a review by Professors Sonnenborn and Proppert. Altogether, these articles surveyed 37 experiments done between 1968 and 1990, involving a total of 2,562 people, with treatments averaging 2 to 3 months. In 13 studies, the participants showed an improvement in mood, and in 11, improvement in intellectual performance. All showed a near-absence of side-effects.

More recent double-blind, controlled trials on ginseng, or ginseng plus ginkgo biloba versus placebos, have proven measurable benefits for energy and memory in both young and old people.[193] Researchers at the Human Cognitive Neuroscience Unit at the University of Northumbria in Newcastle have run three trials, all finding benefit, and are now investigating the herb's precise effect on mental performance.[194]

As with any herb, the dose is critical and ginseng can vary greatly in quality. Good-quality ginseng will state that it is standardised to contain 4 to 7 per cent ginsenosides. The recommended dose of such a standardised extract is 100 to 200mg daily. Ginseng is available as powdered root in capsules or tablets, or as an alcohol-based tincture.

Turmeric – spice up your memory

Turmeric is the bright yellow spice found in most curry powders. You can buy it separately and sprinkle it liberally on your food. Why? Because it reduces joint pain, boosts your immune system and helps prevent Alzheimer's. Turmeric contains the active compound curcumin, which has a variety of powerful anti-inflammatory actions. Trials in which it was given to arthritic patients have shown it to be similarly effective to anti-inflammatory drugs, without the side-effects. Turmeric, as it turns out, is a potent COX 2 enzyme inhibitor, but it does not affect COX 1, which means that you get the pain reduction but not the gastrointestinal side-effects associated with anti-inflammatory drugs. On top of this, it's a potent antioxidant. In fact, in 1995 a patent was filed for turmeric as a 'new' discovery for the treatment of inflammation, but it was rejected after the Indian government challenged the patent on the grounds that turmeric had been used for that very reason for many years in India!

Even more exciting is recent research suggesting that turmeric could help prevent age-related memory loss. Research from the University of California has found that curcumin may be able to break up the 'plaques' that damage the brains of Alzheimer's disease patients. Scientists found that curcumin, the active ingredient within turmeric, was able to reduce deposits of beta-amyloid proteins in the brains of elderly lab mice that ate curcumin as part of their diets.[195]

When researchers added low doses of curcumin to human beta-amyloid proteins in a test tube, the compound kept the proteins from aggregating and blocked the formation of amyloid plaques. 'The new findings suggest that curcumin could be capable of both treating Alzheimer's and lowering a person's risk of developing the disease,' said study co-author Dr Gregory Cole of the University of California Los Angeles.

Huperzia serrata – wave of the future?

Huperzia serrata, or Chinese club moss, has been used for centuries in that country to treat inflammation and fever. More recently, an alkaloid from the herb, huperzine A, has been isolated and developed in China as a licensed drug for the treatment of Alzheimer's.

Huperzine A (also called HupA) is a powerful and highly selective acetylcholinesterase inhibitor, working like the Alzheimer's drug Aricept to keep more acetylcholine in circulation. HupA has shown memory-enhancing effects in clinical trials. Recently it has undergone double-blind, placebo-controlled clinical trials in patients with Alzheimer's disease, with significant improvements both to cognitive function and quality of life. Most of the clinical trials are going on in China.

So far, HupA appears to have fewer side-effects than other acetylcholinesterase inhibitor drugs, such as Aricept, and it may also protect the brain from organophosphates and from too much glutamate (such as the flavouring agent MSG). However, it has also been less thoroughly researched than Aricept.[196]

While HupA is a patented compound, the herb *Huperzia serrata* is not and may therefore be available from herbalists. The recommended daily dose is 200mcg. But note: I would use this herb with caution if at all. It blocks a normal enzyme process and therefore, as with acetylcholinesterase inhibitor drugs, it is likely to have some side-effects; nor does it deal with the underlying cause of low levels of acetylcholine. I feel more research is needed.

Summary: taking herbs for a sharper mind and memory

- Start with 40mg of ginkgo biloba a day and increase up to a maximum of 320mg a day. Choose supplements that use a standardised extract of ginkgo providing about 24 per cent flavonoid content.
- Alternatively, take 10mg of vinpocetine and increase up to a maximum of 40mg a day. Since ginkgo and vinpocetine have similar actions, I don't advise taking both in large amounts.
- Supplement gingseng, 100 to 200mg of a standardised extract containing 4 to 7 per cent ginsenosides.

See Resources, page 251 for details of suppliers of herbal products.

PART 3

Say No to Memory Decline

Whatever your age, you can make an immediate difference to mind, memory and mood by improving your diet, taking the right supplements and making a few simple lifestyle changes. And this plan can carry you through the last third of your life with body and mind in brilliant shape.

17

The Alzheimer's Prevention Diet

ALMOST EVERYTHING WE KNOW about Alzheimer's is pointing clearly to a certain kind of diet, based on a handful of simple principles.

Research at Columbia University Medical Center, New York, has found that those people whose diet includes high intakes of salad dressing, nuts, fish, tomatoes, poultry, fruits, cruciferous vegetables, dark and green leafy vegetables, and low intakes of high-fat dairy, red meat and butter have almost half the risk of developing Alzheimer's.[197]

This diet, consistent with the principles we've discussed, is highly likely both to promote your memory and alertness, whatever your age, and to minimise your chances of heading down the slippery slope towards age-related memory decline and Alzheimer's. I'm aware that some out there would rather adopt a 'wait and see' approach as the evidence accumulates. However, I strongly recommend a more proactive approach. After all, nothing I am going to ask you to do is remotely harmful. In our experience most people start to feel better, and have more consistent mental and physical energy and alertness, within 30 days of starting the Alzheimer's Prevention Diet. This is a good enough reason on its own to take a look at your diet now, and see how it could be changed to a way of eating that will promote your mental and physical health.

The key principles are:

- Eat essential fats and phospholipids.
- Eat slow-release carbohydrates, and avoid refined ones.
- Eat vitamin-, mineral- and antioxidant-rich foods.
- Eat enough protein.
- Avoid harmful fats, refined carbohydrates, sugar and excess caffeine and alcohol.

Now let's see what this means in practice:

Eat essential fats and phospholipids

- Eat an egg a day, or six eggs a week – preferably free range, organic and high in omega-3s. Boil, scramble or poach them, but avoid frying.
- Eat a tablespoon of seeds and nuts every day – the best seeds are flax, hemp, pumpkin, sunflower and sesame. (As for nuts, go for what you like – Brazils, almonds, hazelnuts, cashews...) You get more goodness out of them by grinding them first. They're delicious sprinkled on cereal, soups and salads.
- Eat coldwater, oily carnivorous fish – have a serving of herring, mackerel, salmon or sardines two or three times a week (limit tuna, unless identified as low in mercury, to three times a month).

- Use cold-pressed seed oils – choose an oil blend such as Essential Balance or Udo's Choice for salad dressings and other cold uses, such as drizzling on vegetables instead of butter.

Eat slow-release carbohydrates

- Eat wholefoods – whole grains, lentils, beans, nuts, seeds, fresh fruit and vegetables – and avoid white, refined and over-processed foods.
- Snack on fresh fruit, preferably apples, pears and/or berries.
- Eat four servings a day of whole grains and/or pulses. Try rice, rye, oats, corn, quinoa or wholewheat, boiled or in breads and pasta; and lentils, beans or chickpeas.
- Dilute fruit juices and only eat dried fruit infrequently in small quantities, preferably soaked or with a small handful of nuts or seeds.

Eat antioxidant and vitamin-rich foods

- Eat half your diet raw or lightly steamed.
- Eat three or more servings a day of fresh fruit, including one of berries.
- Eat four servings a day of dark green, leafy and root vegetables such as tenderstem broccoli, broccoli, kale, spinach, watercress, carrots, sweet potatoes, Brussels sprouts, green beans or peppers.
- Have a serving a day of beans, lentils, nuts or seeds – all high in folic acid.

Eat enough protein

- Have three servings of protein-rich foods a day, if you are a man, and two if you are a woman.
- Choose good vegetable protein sources, including beans, lentils, quinoa, tofu or tempeh (soya) and 'seed' vegetables such as peas, broad beans and corn.
- If eating animal protein, choose lean meat or preferably fish, organic whenever possible.

Avoid harmful fats

- Minimise your intake of fried or processed food and saturated fat from meat and dairy products.
- Minimise your consumption of deep-fried food. Poach, steam or steam-fry food instead.

Avoid sugar, reduce caffeine and drink alcohol in moderation

- Avoid adding sugar to dishes, and avoid foods and drinks with added sugar. Keep your sugar intake to a minimum, sweetening cereal or desserts with fruit.
- Avoid or considerably reduce your consumption of caffeinated drinks. Don't have more than one caffeinated drink a day.
- Drink alcoholic drinks infrequently, ideally wine or beer, if your homocysteine score is above 9. Otherwise, have no more than four alcoholic drinks a week.

You may have read the recommendations and realised that much of what you eat falls into the 'avoid' category. If you're wondering how to start making the necessary changes in your shopping, cooking and eating habits, and want help making delicious meals using the principles I outline, read my *Optimum Nutrition Cookbook*.

18

Brain-boosting Supplements

IF YOU WANT TO minimise your risk of developing age-related cognitive decline and Alzheimer's, the Alzheimer's Prevention Diet is a big step in the right direction. But you'll also need to take supplements every day. How much you need to take depends partly on your homocysteine score and partly on your age. If you haven't already tested yourself for homocysteine, now is a good time, so you can build the most appropriate supplement programme for yourself.

The basics

I recommend the following basic daily supplements for everyone:

- **2 x high potency multivitamins and minerals**
- **1 x vitamin C 1000mg**
- **2 x omega-3 and 6 fats**

Multivitamins and minerals

The starting point of any supplement programme is a high-potency multivitamin and multimineral. A good multivitamin should contain at least 2500mcg of vitamin A; 400iu of D; 100iu of E; 250mg of C; 25mg each of B1, B2, B3, B5 and B6; 10mcg of B12; 200mcg of folic acid; and 50mcg of biotin. A good multi-mineral should provide at least 300mg of calcium, 150mg of magnesium, 10mg of iron, 10mg of zinc, 2.5mg of manganese, 20mcg of chromium and 25mcg of selenium, and ideally some molybdenum, vanadium and boron.

You simply can't fit all of the above vitamins and minerals into one tablet. So, as you'll see when you start perusing the labels, with a good combined multivitamin and mineral formula you'll need to take two tablets a day.

Vitamin C

You cannot get enough vitamin C into a decent multivitamin/mineral, so you will need to take this separately. I recommend the equivalent of 1g, plus an additional gram for every two decades above 40. So, if you are 40 plus, take 2g; if you're 60 plus, take 3g; and if you're 80 plus, take 4g. Vitamin C is water soluble and enters and leaves the body within four to six hours. So have your vitamin C in divided doses. If you're taking 3g a day, for example, have 1g with each meal.

Omega-3 and 6 fats

The key essential fats are gamma-linolenic acid (GLA), which is the most potent omega-6 fat; and DHA and EPA, which are the most potent omega-3 fats. I recommend supplementing not less than 300mg of EPA, 200mg of DHA and 100mg of GLA a day. Some supplements provide combinations of omega-3 and 6.

If you are over 60 or suffering from age-related cognitive decline, I recommend doubling the amounts of EPA and DHA to achieve not less than 400mg of both EPA and DHA, or 1000mg of EPA/DHA combined. This is the equivalent of two concentrated omega-3 fish oil capsules a day.

Make sure you buy high-quality essential fat supplements that are effectively guaranteed free from both mercury and PCBs. Companies don't always state this on the packet but a simple phone call should get you a statement or copy of an independent analysis.

Added extras

After you've got to grips with the basics, look to the other brain-boosting nutrients I've discussed in this book:

- **1 x homocysteine formula, if your H score is 7–11.4, or**

  2 x homocysteine formula, if your H score is 11.5–14.9, or

  3 x homocysteine formula, if your H score is above 15
- **1 x antioxidant formula**
- **2 x brain-friendly nutrient formulas**
- **1 x tablespoon of lecithin granules, or a heaped teaspoon of high-PC lecithin a day**
- **Other optional extras**

Homocysteine formula

The first added extra will be homocysteine-lowering nutrients, depending on your H score. Use the chart on page 97 to work out your ideal intake of vitamins B6, B12, folic acid and TMG, based on your H score. A number of supplement companies produce formulas that contain all these. I particularly recommend those that contain methylcobalamin (a form of B12), which appears to be most effective. The best formulas also contain NAC.

Re-test your H score after three months, then lower the amount of homocysteine-busting supplements you are taking.

Antioxidant formula

Everyone can benefit from an all-round antioxidant formula. At the very least, make sure your supplement programme includes 1g of vitamin C, plus 400mg of vitamin E and 20mg of beta-carotene. Ideally, take an all-round antioxidant supplement formula, containing either glutathione or N-acetyl cysteine, co-enzyme Q10 and lipoic acid, plus vitamins A, C and E and the mineral selenium (50mcg). (Acetyl-l-carnitine is an optional extra, but this is generally not in combination antioxidant formulas because the amount you need to make a difference, 250mg, is too bulky.)

As a rule of thumb I would recommend adding an all-round antioxidant formula to your supplement regime once you are over the age of 40, and taking two of these if you are 60 plus, and three of these if you are 80 plus.

Brain-friendly nutrient formulas

Everyone can benefit from brain-friendly nutrients and herbs. These include phosphatidyl choline, phosphatidyl serine, DMAE, pyroglutamate, ginkgo biloba and vinpocetine. (Glutamine is an optional extra, but this is generally not in combination 'brain' formulas because the amount you need to make a difference, 1000mg, is too bulky.) You can find combination brain food supplements that provide many or all of these nutrients. The quantities supplied generally mean that you need two a day.

As a rule of thumb, I would recommend adding two all-round brain-friendly supplements to your regime once you are over the age of 40, and taking three of these if you are 60 plus, and four of these if you are 80 plus.

Lecithin

Even these formulas don't provide an optimal amount of phosphatidyl choline. A good way to boost your intake of phosphatidyl choline is to take lecithin. Some lecithin, called 'Hi PC', is especially high in phosphatidyl choline and hence you won't need so much. I recommend adding a tablespoon of lecithin granules, or a heaped teaspoon of high-PC lecithin a day.

Other optional extras

There is a range of other amino acids, vitamins and herbs that you may need. They include:

- **1 x 250mg of acetyl-l-carnitine, with 120mg of lipoic acid**
- **1000mg of glutamine powder. This is available as a tablet or as a powder, which dissolves in water. Take the equivalent of 1g – half a teaspoon – in water on an empty stomach**
- **1 x niacin 100mg, in addition to the amount in your multivitamin**
- **1 x ginkgo biloba 40mg a day, increasing up to a maximum of 320mg a day. Choose supplements that use a standardised extract of ginkgo, providing about a 24 per cent flavonoid content**

or

- **1 x vinpocetine 10mg, increasing up to a maximum of 40mg a day. Since ginkgo and vinpocetine have similar actions, I don't advise taking both in large amounts**
- **1 x ginseng – 100 to 200mg of a standardised extract containing 4 to 7 per cent ginsenosides**

Aside from the optional extras I discuss above, here's what this all means for you, depending on your age:

The Alzheimer's Prevention Supplement Programme

Supplement	**Under 40**	**40+**	**60+**	**80+**
	Optimum nutrition level			
multivitamin/mineral (see p. 188)	2	2	2	2
Vitamin C 1000mg	1	2	3	4
Omega-3/6 oil capsule	2	2	4	4
Antioxidant formula		1	2	3
Brain nutrient formula		2	3	4
'Hi PC' lecithin			1 teaspoon	1 teaspoon
Homocysteine formula	(depending on your H score)			

But what if...

What if I'm already suffering a decline in memory and concentration?

If you are experiencing poor memory or concentration or age-related cognitive decline, or scored between 18 and 26 on the TICS test (see Appendix 2, page 207), then take the supplements recommended in the table above for the 60 plus age group, even if you are younger than 60.

If you have been diagnosed with dementia, or score less than 18 on the TICS test, take the supplements recommended for the 80 plus age group.

How do I know which specific supplements to take?

I've provided the criteria for choosing each supplement above – particularly the amounts of specific micronutrient they should have. This is almost always at variance with RDA. A supplement may provide 100 per cent of that nutrient's RDA, but such an amount will be much too low to meet the optimal needs of key brain-friendly nutrients.

Also, see the Resources section on page 251 for a list of reputable supplement companies.

How do I know this is safe?

If you're now 80 years old, you'd be taking a lot of supplements under my plan. But even so, the high amounts I recommend are well within the safe upper level for vitamins, minerals and essential fats. (See the next question, however, if you're taking prescribed medication.)

The only real caveat is that you might find yourself getting loose bowels with high amounts of vitamin C. If this happens, just take less. Vitamin A in very large amounts is not recommended in pregnancy. If you are taking three supplements of antioxidant formula – some of which contain vitamin A as retinol – plus a multi, you might be getting too much vitamin A. Of course, if you're 60 or over, you are relatively unlikely to get pregnant! Ginkgo biloba and vinpocetine may thin the blood. Theoretically, this could cause easy bleeding – such as a nosebleed. If this occurs more than once, reduce the amount you take.

Can I take these nutrients with prescribed medication?

Don't take ginkgo biloba or vinpocetine if you are on blood-thinning drugs (aspirin or warfarin) without discussing the idea with your doctor. I am unaware of any other potential drug-nutrient interactions. But just to be on the safe side, I would recommend asking your doctor to confirm there are no contraindicated nutrients if you are on prescribed drugs. Folic acid, for example, is not recommended for people taking some anti-epilepsy drugs.

If I need help, who can I ask?

Come to the Brain Bio Centre for a full assessment of your cognitive health, including all the biochemical tests referred to in this book. The centre is the clinical division of the Food for the Brain Foundation, an educational charity. (You can find out more at www.brainbiocentre.com.) Their staff include psychiatrists and nutritional therapists who specialise in age-related memory loss and dementia/Alzheimer's disease. I also have a team of highly qualified clinical nutritionists throughout Britain, and abroad. They can offer personal nutrition consultations and can support you with your nutritional regime. To find out details of the nutritional therapists nearest to you go to www.patrickholford.com and select 'Find a nutritionist' in the 'advice' section.

How do I know it's working? How long do I take these supplements?

Monitor your results using 'Your Brain MOT' in Appendix 1. For this you'll need to fill in some of the questionnaires in this book again. Also, re-test your homocysteine level. Most people start to feel areas of improvement within three months.

Rather than sticking rigidly to my supplement recommendations, you may wish to try adding or taking away something and noticing any difference. I do not, however, recommend you ever stop taking the basics (see page 187). Nor do I recommend you stop taking the homocysteine-lowering nutrients I list until your homocysteine score is under control.

19

Exercises to Keep Your Mind Sharp

WITH THE RIGHT NUTRITION and the right attitude, age-related memory loss doesn't need to happen to you. You can build new brain cells at any age. Research clearly shows that healthy, well-educated elderly people can show no decline in mental function right up to death, and no increased rate of brain shrinkage even after 65. There is also plenty of evidence that keeping both your mind and body active will help to prevent a decline in mental function.[198–203]

Use it – or lose it

For example, researchers at the Albert Einstein College of Medicine in New York have tested the link between leisure activities and the risk of developing dementia or Alzheimer's disease in the elderly. They studied 469 people over the age of 75 who had no signs of dementia at the start. Following them over a period of five years, the team found that reading, playing cards and board games, doing crossword puzzles, playing musical instruments and dancing were all associated with a reduced risk of dementia, memory loss and Alzheimer's disease. Overall, the study participants who did these kinds of activities about four days a week were two-thirds less likely to get Alzheimer's, compared with those who did these activities once a week or less.[204]

Researchers at the Rush Alzheimer's Disease Center in Chicago found the same things when they studied a group of 801 Catholic nuns and priests who had no signs of dementia over four and a half years. They compared the amount of mentally stimulating activity each person engaged in and measured their rate of mental decline, and found that increased mental activity was associated with a reduced decline in overall mental function by 47 per cent, memory by 60 per cent, and perception by 30 per cent.[205]

Keep fit

Your cognitive powers aren't all that need exercising. Getting your body into gear has a direct effect on your mind, memory and mood, for a number of reasons.

First, there's the fact that the brain and body are largely made of the same stuff, and since we know that exercise keeps your body healthy, it stands to reason that it will keep your brain healthy, too. Secondly, part of the benefit of exercise is that it helps reduce stress, and as we saw in Chapter 14, stress rapidly ages the brain. Thirdly, exercise increases the flow of blood to the brain, bringing more oxygen and nutrients with it.[206–7] It has even been shown to increase the size of your brain.[208] And lastly, there is evidence that being overweight and at greater risk of cardiovascular disease increase the risk of Alzheimer's, so those dividends of exercise – lower weight and better cardio health – have a knock-on effect on the brain.

Both exercising and just keeping active make a big difference. For example, people who participate in leisure-time physical activity that lasts at least 20 to 30 minutes, and causes breathlessness and sweating, twice a week or more cut their risk of age-related memory decline by a staggering 65 per cent![209] Evidence for the importance of keeping fit was also found in a five-year study of 5,000 Canadian men and women over the age of 65. Those who kept up high levels of physical activity, compared to those who rarely exercised, halved their risk of Alzheimer's disease.[210] Another study in the US also found a halving of risk in those who exercised three times a week.[211]

One study found that regular walking improved memory and reduced signs of dementia: about 1,000 steps, or a little over a mile a day, was the minimum distance required to achieve the positive effect.[212] Yet another study, this time conducted in Italy, found that among a group of 65 year olds without memory problems, those in the top third of activity had a quarter of the risk of developing Alzheimer's compared to those in the bottom third.[213]

More recently, the potential benefits of exercise were put to the test in a controlled trial in which people with age-related memory decline, but not dementia, were assigned to a 24–week home-based physical activity regime or a 'usual care' group. Those in the exercise group had improvements in memory tests, while those in the 'usual care' group had a decline in their memory function.[214] So the moral of this story is to keep active.

Exercise, it seems, also prevents physical deterioration of the brain. Our brains become less dense and lose volume as we age, and with that loss of density and volume comes mental decline. Researchers at the University of Illinois used MRI scans to examine the brains of 55 elderly people. When they compared the scans with the individuals' level of physical activity, they found that the people who exercised more and were more physically fit had the densest brains.[215] So – if you don't use your body, you could lose your mind.

Exercise not only protects against Alzheimer's, it can also lift your mood. In fact, it's more effective than antidepressants for mild depression. Depression is a common problem among Alzheimer's patients. A study at the University of Washington in Seattle showed that exercise significantly improved the mood and physical health of depressed Alzheimer's patients, and meant they were less likely to need to be moved into a care home.[216]

Stay trim

Maintaining the right weight for your build also reduces your risk. A Swedish study found that being overweight increases the risk of Alzheimer's. Studying 392 men and women for 18 years, the researchers found that the overweight women had a much higher rate of Alzheimer's. For every 1 point increase in body mass index (BMI, calculated by taking your weight in kilograms and dividing it by your height in metres squared) at the age of 70, the risk of Alzheimer's increased by over a third. Oddly enough, they didn't find the same result in men.[217]

Breathe deep...

Since oxygen is the brain's most vital nutrient, learning to breathe more fully is likely to help keep your mind young. Breathing techniques are fundamental to all types of yoga and also many of the martial arts.

A type of breathing used in the practice of yoga, which involves breathing through one or other nostril or alternate nostrils, has been studied by two groups of researchers to see if there was any impact on memory. Both groups found that this type of breathing improved 'spatial' but not verbal memory.[218–19] Spatial memory is the type of memory you would use to find your car in the car park. There may be other benefits to yoga, since it reduces stress, increases blood flow to the brain and improves physical fitness.

I strongly recommend you take up yoga, t'ai chi, qigong or other similar activities that help you develop both breathing and centring techniques as well as fitness. These also help to reduce your stress levels.

One of my favourite exercise routines is Psychocalisthenics.® Psychocalisthenics is a precise sequence of 23 exercises that leave you feeling fantastic. I've been doing it for over 20 years and I've yet to find anything that keeps me trimmer and makes me feel better – which isn't bad for 15 minutes a day! Each exercise is driven by the breath and, somehow, my body feels lighter, freer and thoroughly oxygenated after this simple routine, which anyone can do.

Psychocalisthenics is the brainchild of Oscar Ichazo, who founded the Arica School in the 1960s as a school of knowledge for the understanding of the complete person. A practitioner of martial arts and yoga since 1939, he developed Psychocalisthenics as a daily routine that can be done in less than 20 minutes. At first glance, it looks like a kind of aerobic yoga. 'In the same way that we have an everyday need for food and nourishment we have to promote the circulation of our vital energy as an everyday business,' says Ichazo.

While most exercise routines simply treat the body as a physical machine that needs to be worked to stay fit, Psychocalisthenics is designed to generate both physical fitness and vital energy by bringing mind and body into balance. The key lies in the precise breathing pattern that accompanies each physical exercise. Energy generation happens when you have stable blood sugar, plus a good supply of oxygen. According to Jane Alexander of the *Daily Mail*, 'Psychocalisthenics is exercise, pared to perfection. I wasn't sweating buckets as I would after an aerobics class. But I had exercised far more muscles. I was clear-headed and bright rather than wiped out.'

The best way to learn Psychocalisthenics is to do a short course. For details see www.patrickholford.com/psychocalisthenics. You can also teach yourself from a DVD, but it is best to learn it 'live'. See Resources on page 250 for information on Psychocalisthenics and finding classes in yoga or t'ai chi.

Learn to meditate

Although there's no substantial research on the effects of meditation for the prevention of memory loss, meditation is the ultimate antidote to the effects of stress on every level. Physically, it reduces heart rate and blood pressure, slows the rate of breathing and stabilises brain wave patterns. It also improves the body's responsiveness to stressful events and aids quicker recovery – and has been shown to prevent the depression of the body's immune responses that occurs with stress.

The benefits of meditation on mental and emotional health are far-reaching. There's no doubt that meditation helps dissolve anxiety and promotes clarity and peace of mind. In fact, people who practise meditation on a regular basis have been found to be less anxious, and research has found that meditators have lower levels of the stress hormone cortisol. And as we saw in Chapter 14, the harmful effects of cortisol on the brain are such that reducing it is of paramount importance.

What meditation offers is, in fact, no small thing. Although we cannot change what happens to us from day to day, we can change the way we respond to stressful situations. Regular meditation helps us become less reactive to the normal stresses and strains of life, so that we can sustain a happy, relaxed state of mind.

Most meditation techniques involve focusing on one object as a way to calm the mind. This object could be repetition of a mantra (such as 'Om'), the flame of a candle, or the breath.

Research at the Heffter Research Institute in Santa Fe, New Mexico (see www.heffter.org), on the effects of focusing on the breath suggests that this helps bring the brain into balance. With this balance comes a sense of connection, clarity and happiness. As the mind quietens, your powers of concentration and mental agility improve. You are more able to focus your energy on the task at hand, instead of dissipating energy by trying to 'multitask' without doing any individual task completely.

Meditation is much like physical exercise: it is more beneficial to meditate for 10 minutes every day than to meditate for an hour once a week. Daily practice – even if it's only for a few minutes – will quickly get your mind into the habit of meditating. Just like physical exercise, the more you do it, the easier it gets.

When you first start meditating, give yourself a realistic timeframe. Start with at least 10 minutes every day. As your mind and body get used to those 10 minutes, increase the time to 15 minutes and so on. There is no time limit to meditation, but see what feels best for you. The best thing to do is to find a course that can teach you to meditate, then build it into your daily routine.

Let there be light

Vitamins, minerals, amino acids and so forth aside, one of the brain's 'nutrients' is light. Light helps stimulate the production of neurotransmitters in the brain. In fact, you wake up because light enters through the eyelids – which are thin-skinned enough to admit it – and the translucent portions of the skull; this triggers the production of adrenalin, which 'jogs' you awake. Light also promotes healthy levels of serotonin.

So light therapy has had promising results for people with memory loss. A study looking into light therapy as a way of improving memory was carried out at the University of Vienna in Austria. Alzheimer's patients who took part in the study had significantly better scores on memory tests following 'bright light therapy', compared with using dim light.[220]

In this kind of therapy, you sit near a special light box fitted with high-intensity light bulbs, which provide full-spectrum or white light with a capacity of 10,000 lux (the international unit of illumination – 1 lumen per square metre). This type of light is about 15 times brighter than normal home or office lighting. You can buy light boxes such as these for your home as well as 'full-spectrum' light bulbs that fit into a standard light bulb fitting. My advice is to invest in a full-spectrum 'reading' light and have this on whenever you can. Also fit full-spectrum light bulbs in the places you spend the most time, whether the office, the living room or kitchen. Additionally, get outside in natural daylight as much as you can.

And keep discovering...

Other complementary or alternative therapies such as reflexology, music and singing are likely to be beneficial for mental health for the same reasons as the other physically and mentally stimulating activities mentioned above. They have not been thoroughly investigated but since they are safe and enjoyable, why not give them a try too!

Summary: making simple lifestyle changes to keep your mind young

- Learn new skills and engage in mentally stimulating activities such as games, puzzles and crosswords frequently.
- Play, listen to and dance to music as much as you can.
- Keep as physically active as possible with exercise. If walking is your exercise, walk a mile a day. Ideally, take up an exercise that helps develop 'yogic' breathing, such as yoga, t'ai chi or Psychocalisthenics.
- Learn to meditate. There are simple courses available.
- Make sure you get enough light. Spend some time outdoors most days. Use full-spectrum lighting. Have a sunny holiday in winter.

Appendix 1: Your Brain's MOT

So you can keep a record of how you are now, and how your mental health changes over the next three to six months, complete your scores from the questionnaires in this book in the form below.

Name:

Today's date: __/__/__ 3 Months: __/__/__ 6 Months: __/__/__

Your TICS Test score (see Appendix 2)

Your score: ___ Your score: ___ Your score: ___

Your Mind and Memory Check (page 8)

Your score: ___ Your score: ___ Your score: ___

Alzheimer's Risk Factor Check (page 38)

Your score: ___ Your score: ___ Your score: ___

Neurotransmitter Checks (page 44)

Your score for		
Acetylcholine: ___	Your score: ___	Your score: ___
Serotonin: ___	Your score: ___	Your score: ___
Dopamine: ___	Your score: ___	Your score: ___
GABA: ___	Your score: ___	Your score: ___

Essential Brain Foods Checks (Chapter 6)

Your score for		
Essential Fats: ___	Your score: ___	Your score: ___
Phospholipids: ___	Your score: ___	Your score: ___
Amino acids: ___	Your score: ___	Your score: ___
Intelligent nutrients: ___	Your score: ___	Your score: ___

Appendix 2: Test Your Memory

DO NOT TURN OVER THIS PAGE

On the next page is a simple test called the Telephone Interview for Cognitive Status (TICS) test. This test is only valid if someone else asks you the questions in person, or by phone. The procedure is very simple, but only valid if you have not seen the questions.

Please find someone to administer this test to you, then add up your score.

Telephone Interview for Cognitive Status (TICS-M)

Score 1 for each correct answer and 0 if incorrect.

Questions	*Answers*	
Orientation		
1 (i) What day of the week is it?	Day	______
(ii) What is today's date?	Date	______
	Month	______
	Year	______
(ii) What season are we in?	Season	______
2 What is your age?	Age	______
3 What is your telephone number? (code and number)	______	

Registration/Free Recall

4 I'm going to read you a list of 10 words. Please listen carefully and try to remember them. When I am done, tell me as many as you can in any order. Ready?

Cabin
Pipe
Elephant
Chest
Silk
Theatre
Watch
Whip
Pillow
Giant

Now, tell me all the words you can remember. ______

______

______

Attention/Calculation

5	Please take 7 away from 100 Now continue to take 7 away from what you have left over until I ask you to stop.	☐ 93
		☐ 86
		☐ 79
		☐ 72
		☐ 65
6	Please count backwards from 20 to 1.	☐ no mistakes

Comprehension, Semantic and Recent Memory

7	What do people usually use to cut paper?	☐ Scissors
8	What is the prickly green plant found in the desert?	☐ Cactus
9	Who is the reigning monarch now?	☐ E, QE, QE2
10	Who is the Prime Minister now?	☐ Correct surname
11	What is the opposite of east?	☐ West

Language/Repetition

12	Please say this 'Methodist Episcopal'.	☐ Exactly right

Delayed Recall

13	Please repeat the list of 10 words I read earlier.	☐ Cabin
		☐ Pipe
		☐ Elephant
		☐ Chest
		☐ Silk
		☐ Theatre
		☐ Watch
		☐ Whip
		☐ Pillow
		☐ Giant
		Add up – maximum of 39 ☐

Interpreting your score:

27 or more indicates that you are not experiencing significant cognitive decline.

18–26 indicates a degree of cognitive impairment. We recommend that you see your doctor as well as following the recommendations in this book.

Less than 18 indicates serious cognitive impairment. We recommend that you see your doctor as well as following the recommendations in this book.

Appendix 3: Success Stories

In this appendix I relate some of the success stories of people with cognitive decline, diagnosed dementia or Alzheimer's disease, who have either made a recovery, or stopped getting any worse. Let's kick off with one of the pioneers of positive thinking – and action – in the field, who knows from the inside out that recovery is possible.

Tom Warren

Now in his seventies, Tom was diagnosed with Alzheimer's at the age of 50.

Case study

At 47, my memory started to decline. I had a difficult time finding my car in parking lots. Sometimes I couldn't remember my own telephone number. I was in a perpetual fog, confused, disoriented and became a crabby obnoxious idiot. Eventually I couldn't do my job and was fired.

In June 1983, at the age of 50, our family doctor sent me to St Peter Hospital, in Olympia, Washington, for a CAT scan. The next day my doctor told me I had Alzheimer's and said that I might have as long as seven years to live. A few days later another doctor rechecked my X-rays and pointed out the brain atrophy revealed by the CAT scan and said there was no doubt about the accuracy of the diagnosis.

I felt as if I was standing off in the fog knowing that things are going on just beyond your reach you can't do anything about. I was so exhausted it would have been so very easy to lie down, to rest, to die. I'm not able to make myself think more about that time. It's too painful.

Today I am almost completely well. My thought process has diminished a bit, but on the whole I feel well and my memory is just fine. I have finished writing my second book and am working on a third.

If you or a loved one have chronic disease, especially schizophrenia, Alzheimer's, dementia or other neurological disorders such as MS that your doctor does not know the underlying cause for and you are not getting well, look in your mouth. My turning point came when I had 26 mercury fillings removed. Do not go to any dentist who still places silver/mercury amalgam fillings or does root canals. Fifteen years ago dentists might not have known how dangerous amalgam fillings and root canals really are.

Find a good environmental doctor. Find out about your own allergies and chemical sensitivities. Work with a nutritionist. Learn about nutrition. Take a comprehensive supplement programme including vitamin B3, B6, and folic acid. Get some really good advice on vitamins, minerals and supplements. To be honest, I don't know one single person who followed this advice and did not get better.

Tom Warren has written two books that may be of interest to sufferers and their families: Beating Alzheimer's *and* Reversing Chronic Disease *(see Recommended Reading page 245).*

Tom Warrren's story is only one of the more dramatic in the context of recovery from dementia. As the relevance of optimum nutrition to mental and emotional health is recognised more and more, the success stories are piling up. Let's look at some of these case studies.

Case study

Lilly began to suffer from a deteriorating memory in her mid-sixties. At 70 she was finally diagnosed with Alzheimer's. She became progressively disorientated, forgetful, disturbed and unhappy. She realised something was wrong with her brain but refused any overt medical help.

Within two years, Lilly required a level of care that could no longer be provided at home, so her husband reluctantly moved her into a nursing home. He, meanwhile, began researching the available literature on Alzheimer's and came across Patrick Holford's *Optimum Nutrition for the Mind*. He worked with a qualified nutritionist to devise a diet and supplement programme for Lilly along the lines of the Alzheimer's Prevention Plan, which was implemented with the approval of Lilly's consultant and the cooperation of the nursing home staff.

Within 10 weeks Lilly was showing small but encouraging improvements in memory, so her husband decided to contact the Brain Bio Centre in London. After a series of blood tests and consultations, a supplement programme was devised for Lilly to take account of the test results, which revealed food allergies, neurotransmitter deficiencies and raised homocysteine levels. Within a few weeks, Lilly's husband, her sons and several friends noticed continuing significant improvements in her short and long-term memories, responsiveness, awareness and lucidity.

Case study

Virginia began to experience a decline in memory and concentration in her early seventies. She also found herself becoming quite irritable. At the age of 77, she consulted the Brain Bio Centre in London, which ran tests that showed neurotransmitter and mineral imbalances. She was advised to include more seeds and nuts in her diet, reduce the amount of coffee she was drinking, and supplement extra nutrients, including fish oils and antioxidants. Within a few months, Virginia was feeling much brighter and less sleepy. Her daughter noticed that she had better recollection of what she had been doing from day to day and was generally more positive and less irritable. Virginia's balance and joints, which had been bothering her, also improved.

Case study

Claire first visited her GP complaining of problems with her short-term memory, which had been bothering her over the previous year. She was 70. At this stage no diagnosis or treatment was given. Over the following 18 months, her memory continued to decline steadily, so she visited her doctor again. The doctor diagnosed 'age-associated memory impairment' and gave her a test which showed that her memory was poor, but offered no treatment.

Eighteen months after this, both she and her husband felt that her memory had got much worse. She had begun asking her husband inappropriate questions and was struggling with general day-to-day tasks. A repeat of the memory test showed that her memory had indeed declined significantly over the preceding 18 months.

She was prescribed a medication that is designed to help with memory in such cases, an acetylcholinesterase inhibitor that is the 'gold-standard' treatment for people suffering with age-related memory decline. Since the medication didn't seem to be helping at all and she found its side-effects unpleasant, she stopped the medication after a few weeks.

Folic acid supplements were prescribed some months later, but these didn't seem to help either. A test showed that her blood levels of B12 were low, so she began to have monthly B12 injections. Again no improvement was seen over the next six months. Because her blood levels of glutathione (an antioxidant) were also shown to be low in tests, a daily dose of N-acetyl cysteine (NAC) was prescribed. (As we saw in the case of Mary, glutathione can be made in the body from NAC, and glutathione can make the body use vitamin B12 more effectively.)

Within one month of starting the NAC she had improved dramatically. Her husband noticed that she was much livelier, happier and chattier and her practice nurse said that for the first time in many months she could hold a sensible conversation and that her general behaviour had improved. The memory test was re-run and confirmed that there had been a marked improvement in her memory.

Case study

Rebecca visited her GP complaining of losing her memory and feeling confused over the past several months. She was particulary concerned because she had an aunt who suffered from early-onset Alzheimer's. The doctor found that she did indeed have considerable problems with her memory and ran some tests. A blood test revealed that she was low in vitamin

B12, so he prescribed monthly injections. Over the next two years, however, Rebecca's memory continued to get worse and she became increasingly fatigued and unwell. She also began to suffer visual hallucinations and irrational fears of persecution. Mental testing showed that while her short-term memory was very poor and she was disorientated in terms of time, her memory of the distant past was quite reasonable. She had also begun experiencing problems with coordination, which affected her handwriting. She was diagnosed with 'probable Alzheimer's' and admitted to a nursing home.

There, tests confirmed that her mental function continued to decline. At this time, she was prescribed an acetylcholinesterase inhibitor, the most common treatment for people suffering from age-related memory decline. Her family felt that she improved somewhat initially. However, her physical and mental health continued to decline steadily, and seven years on from her initial visit to her doctor she had 'severe dementia'.

At this point, she was prescribed a daily dose of N-acetyl cysteine (NAC), in addition to the vitamin B12 injections and the acetylcholinesterase inhibitor. The nursing home staff and her family noticed a 'significant' improvement: she became brighter, more alert and seemed to recognise her close family. Sadly, she died of pneumonia several weeks later.

Case study

Frank consulted his GP complaining that his memory had been steadily worsening over the past three years. His doctor found no other symptoms of disease but did find a degree of deterioration in both recent and past memory. All blood tests came back normal with the exception of homocysteine, which was quite high. A CT brain scan showed some shrinkage of the brain but no other problems. He was given a diagnosis of 'probable Alzheimer's'.

Because of the high homocysteine level found in his blood, which can be a factor in dementia, monthly injections of B12 and daily doses of folic acid were prescribed, even though his levels of these vitamins tested normal. Over the next three years his mental function continued to deteriorate until at last he was admitted to a nursing home.

He was not prescribed medication for the dementia because the disease was already at such an advanced stage. His mental function continued to decline steadily and this was confirmed by repeat mental tests two years later. At this point his homocysteine level was normal, but tests showed his levels of the antioxidant glutathione were very low. He was prescribed a daily dose of N-acetyl cysteine (NAC) to help raise the level of glutathione. The staff at the nursing home and Frank's wife noticed a significant improvement in his behaviour and communication. He now seemed to recognise his wife when she visited and actually attempted communication with her for the first time in many years. The improvement was still continuing a year later.

Appendix 4: Drugs and Hormones – The Best and the Worst

The current medications for dementia and Alzheimer's are somewhat limited and don't really deal with the underlying causes of the neuronal damage. What they do is boost the brain's levels of acetylcholine, the memory neurotransmitter. This produces improvement in about 20 per cent of people, but only as long as they have enough neurons. Once the disease progresses, however, the drugs rapidly stop working.

The main Alzheimer's drugs

There are two main classes of drugs used to treat Alzheimer's: the acetylcholinesterase inhibitors, including donepezil (Aricept), rivastigmine (Exelon), and galantamine (Reminyl); and a newer drug called memantine (Namenda).

The acetylcholinesterase inhibitors prevent an enzyme known as acetylcholinesterase from breaking down acetylcholine in the brain. Increased concentrations of acetylcholine lead to a boost in communication between nerve cells, which may in turn temporarily improve or stabilise the symptoms of Alzheimer's disease in about a fifth of patients, as we've seen. However, when the drug is withdrawn, people tend to deteriorate rapidly over a period of about four to six weeks, until they are no better than someone who has never taken the drug. One reason why the effects of these drugs don't last is that they don't address the underlying cause of the disease, namely neuronal degeneration.

The most widely prescribed of these drugs is Aricept. The longest trial of Aricept (lasting five years) was recently published in the *Lancet*, and researchers found no difference in 'worthwhile improvements', including rates of disease progression, the rate at which people with Alzheimer's were placed in nursing homes, caregiver time, or behaviour decline – regardless of the dosage given. However, during the first two years of the study, patients taking Aricept did do slightly better in tests gauging thinking and functional ability. Even the study's lead researcher, Richard Gray, admitted, 'Realistically, patients are unlikely to derive much benefit from this drug.'[221]

Memantine works in a different way. High homocysteine makes your brain's neurons more susceptible to damage from a naturally occurring neurotransmitter called glutamate, which causes over-excitation and neuronal death. Memantine can protect brain cells by blocking the receptor, the docking port, for glutamate. While it helps some people with raised homocysteine, the safer alternative is to lower homocysteine levels with B vitamins.

Side-effects of acetylcholinesterase inhibitors include nausea, vomiting, diarrhoea, stomach cramps, headaches, dizziness, fatigue, insomnia, and loss of appetite.

The side-effects of memantine include hallucinations, confusion, dizziness, headaches and tiredness.

Another drug that is sometimes used is Deprenyl. Also called Selegiline, it is one of a group of drugs called mono-amino-oxidase inhibitors, or MAOIs for short. They work as antidepressants by preventing neurotransmitters from being broken down. Most of these drugs, however, are associated with potentially dangerous side-effects; they're known as MAO-A inhibitors. Deprenyl, on the other hand, is much safer, since it is an MAO-B inhibitor.[222]

Deprenyl is particularly effective at halting the breakdown of dopamine, a deficiency of which is associated with Parkinson's disease. It is mainly prescribed for treating both Parkinson's and Alzheimer's disease. Some people recommend taking it to prevent these diseases and as a general stimulant to mental functioning, even when no symptoms are present. In animals it has also been shown to extend lifespan.[223]

Research by the National Institutes of Health in the US has shown that 10mg of Deprenyl does significantly improve memory, attention span and learning in people with Alzheimer's.[224] To what extent it makes a difference in normal people is a subject of controversy. If you want to try taking it, start with 1 or 2mg and build up to 5mg. If you experience insomnia, lower the dose. Deprenyl is available on prescription as Eldepryl, but the liquid form (Deprenyl citrate) can be ordered by post.

Enter the smart drug

None of these drugs is suitable for preventing Alzheimer's. However, over 100 'smart drugs' have already been developed, and once 'age-related memory decline' becomes a classifiable disease, there is no doubt that such drugs will become very widely used in society. Some have also been shown to enhance mental abilities in those without diagnosed memory problems. This raises the important question of whether some of these drugs should be used to help prevent these, and even promote memory and concentration in those without cognitive problems, or whether their use should be restricted to those with cognitive problems.

For the pharmaceuticals industry, the advantage of these drugs is that they are not nutrients but in most cases man-made substances – that is, they can be patented and hence are more profitable. But for us, they have a major disadvantage: they are alien to the human body. They may not produce a 'perfect fit' in enzyme systems, and while creating the desired effect in the short term, they may, in the long term, unbalance the brain's sensitive chemistry. In any case, with many of these new smart drugs, the long-term effects are still unknown. So it is best to proceed with caution.

Smart drugs for Alzheimer's fall into one of two categories:

- Drugs that mimic or improve the action of neurotransmitters. These include Piracetam and Hydergine.
- Hormones that influence brain function. These include DHEA and pregnenolone.

These are by no means the only smart drugs and hormones used for Alzheimer's, but they are among the most interesting, well researched and widely taken, with a track record of relative safety. They therefore have a potential role in restoring an active memory and mind.

However, as attractive as smart drugs and hormones might seem, my recommendation is not to take them, at least not in the first instance. In many cases, the combination of mind- and memory-enhancing nutrients does the trick. However, if these steps alone do not produce the effect you are after, and you suffer from the conditions listed overleaf, you may wish to experiment with the following smart drugs and hormones – but only under the guidance of your doctor or a suitably qualified health practitioner.

No matter what your circumstances, my recommendation is to start with no more than one smart drug or hormone, at the lower dose (with the exception of Piracetam), and build up gradually, noting how you respond, and stopping at the dose that produces the best results for you. Then add others as required. But remember: please check with your doctor before taking any of these drugs or hormones.

Smart Drugs, Smart Hormones

Symptom	Drug/hormone	Dose
Pronounced memory loss, dementia or Alzheimer's		
	Hydergine	9mg
	Piracetam	4800mg
	Pregnenolone	25mg
	DHEA	15mg

It has also been found that taking smart drugs with 'smart nutrients' such as phosphatidyl choline, pantothenic acid, DMAE and pyroglutamate boosts the drug's efficacy. In a study in 1981, a team of researchers led by Raymond Bartus gave choline and Piracetam to aged lab rats noted for age-related memory decline.[225] Their finding was that rats given this combination had memory retention scores several times better than those taking Piracetam alone. Results also showed that half the dose was needed when Piracetam and choline were combined. Some 'brain food' supplements contain combinations of all these acetylcholine-friendly nutrients – choline, DMAE, pantothenic acid and pyroglutamate.

Now let's take a closer look at how some smart drugs work, and what side-effects they might have.

The lowdown on smart drugs

Piracetam is one of a number of drugs called 'nootropics', which are related to the amino acid pyroglutamate. Over 150 studies have been published on Piracetam, which has been shown to enhance mental performance on a number of counts. Numerous studies have shown improvements in memory, concentration, coordination and reaction time.[226] The drug appears more effective in the early stages of memory decline.

Studies using Piracetam have demonstrated clear improvements in memory, mood and cognitive abilities in both animals and humans.[227] One such study tested the effects of Piracetam on 18 people aged 50 and older, with demanding jobs and above-average IQs, who were basically fully functional except that they were having problems retaining and recalling memory.

They were extensively tested for cognitive function and assigned to the Piracetam or placebo group, without them or the researchers knowing who was on the real thing. On re-testing those taking Piracetam, their performance on a number of cognitive tests had significantly improved. These people were then put on placebo, while those previously on placebo were given Piracetam. Again, the Piracetam group improved dramatically while those on the placebo did not.[228]

Another double-blind placebo-controlled trial involved 162 French people aged 55 and over with age-related memory decline who had sought help from their doctor. The group taking Piracetam showed beneficial effects after just six weeks.[229]

These are just a couple of several convincing studies that have led to Piracetam being widely prescribed. Nootropil, one brand of Piracetam, has had registered sales of over US$1 billion in recent years.

Piracetam seems to promote memory retention, improve acetylcholine transmission and reception, reduce the effects of stress and speed up reaction time. The question is, how? Part of its mode of action is that it improves communication across the corpus callosum, which connects the two hemispheres of the brain. Thus it improves the link between our analytical and relational thinking processes, which is most helpful for storing and finding memories. One study, published in 1988 by doctors H. Pilch and W. E. Muller, found that mice given Piracetam for two weeks had 30 to 40 per cent more acetylcholine receptors than before.[230] This suggests that pyroglutamate-like molecules may also have a regenerative effect on the nervous system. The weight of evidence seems to show, then, that this nutrient-like drug is well worth considering for those with Alzheimer's.

And all the more so because Piracetam is, by all accounts, very safe and has no side-effects at effective doses. It usually comes in 800mg capsules, and the recommended dose is three to six capsules per day (2400 to 4800mg). Since positive effects may only occur at higher doses, my recommendation is to start with 4800mg for two weeks, then reduce the dose back to 2400mg or whatever level continues to be effective. Remember, Piracetam is far more effective if given with choline. The drug is available on prescription in the US, or without prescription outside the US.

Hydergine is the most widely used and thoroughly tested prescription drug for improving brain function. Its scientific name is ergoloid mesylate, and it is an extract of the ergot fungus that grows on rye and was discovered in the 1950s by Albert Hoffman (better known for his discovery of that other ergot-based drug, LSD). It works by improving circulation to the brain and protecting against oxidant damage. It also seems to improve the production of neurotransmitters, especially dopamine, noradrenalin and acetylcholine, and stabilises the brain's glucose metabolism. In 1994 researchers from the University of California reviewed the results of 47 trials testing Hydergine for its effects on reversing memory loss in those with dementia. The majority of these studies showed that it is effective, although it was little help for those with Alzheimer's.[231]

But there is some evidence that Hydergine improves memory in healthy people. In a UK study, 12 volunteers without cognitive problems were given cognitive tests before and after receiving 12mg of Hydergine for two weeks. The results showed significant improvement in their alertness and cognitive abilities.[232]

The usual dose for Hydergine is 9mg, given as 3mg three times a day. It appears to be non-toxic, although there are rare reports of nausea and headaches. If that happens, stop taking it.

The lowdown on memory-boosting hormones

One step closer to nature than smart drugs are the 'smart hormones'. These are naturally occurring hormones that have an effect on our mental performance. In this category come pregnenolone and DHEA. In the US, these natural hormones are sold over the counter to deal with anything from jet lag to extending life. In the UK and most other countries, they are only available on prescription.

DHEA and **pregnenolone** are naturally occurring hormones, but that certainly doesn't make them harmless. As you can see in Figure 18 overleaf, they can, if needed, be turned into oestrogen and testosterone. Pregnenolone can also be transformed into progesterone and adrenal hormones. So they can have a powerful effect on the balance of sex hormones, as well as adrenal hormones, which are involved in the stress response. Low levels of oestrogen, progesterone and adrenal hormones are all associated with declining memory. However, attempting to correct these with conventional HRT (oestrogen plus progestins) is more likely to increase your risk for dementia, not reverse it.[233]

Both DHEA and pregnenolone levels tend to decrease with age, and the simplistic view is that topping them up will stop the ageing process. The trouble is, having more than you need means the body has to work hard to get rid of the excess. So for these hormones, more is not necessarily better. While potentially useful

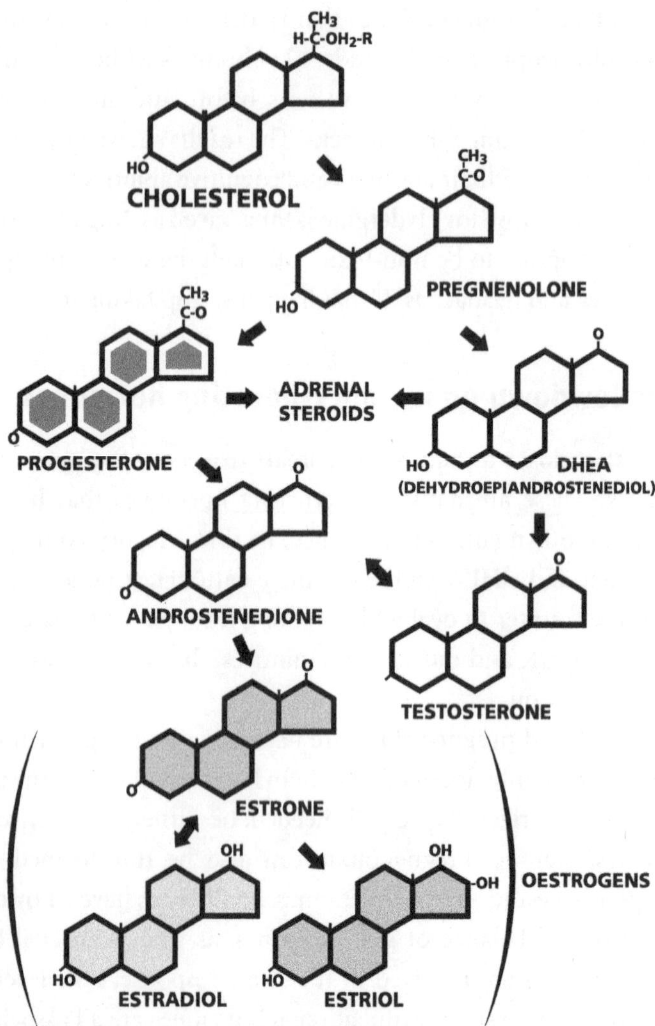

Figure 18. The hormone family tree. All steroid hormones are made from cholesterol. One way arrows denote one way conversion. For example, progesterone can be turned into adrenal steroids, testosterone and oestrogens, but oestrogens cannot be turned into progesterone

for those with adrenal exhaustion, blood sugar problems and hormonal imbalances, they are not recommended for supplementation except under the guidance of a health practitioner.

'Before and after' tests should be carried out to determine whether or not there is a deficiency, in which case correcting it is likely to improve mental functioning. The older you are, the more likely you are to have low levels of DHEA and pregnenolone. For this reason, many older people in the US supplement up to 25mg of pregnenolone or 15mg of DHEA a day. More than this is unwise without proper testing. DHEA and pregnenolone should be taken in the morning, before breakfast.

References and Resources

References

1 Kalaria R. et al., 'Alzheimer's disease and vascular dementia in developing countries: prevalence, management, and risk factors', *Lancet Neurology*, 7:812–26 (2008).

2 Wimo A. et al., 'The magnitude of dementia occurrence in the world', *Alzheimers Disease and Associated Disorders*, 17(2):63–7 (2003).

3 100% Health Survey, see www.patrickholford.com/100survey

4 Rowe J.W., Kahn R.L.,'Human aging: usual and successful', *Science*, 237(4811):143–9 (1987); and Schaie K.W., 'The Seattle Longitudinal Study: A thirty-five-year inquiry of adult intellectual development', *Z Gerontol*, 26(3):129–37 (1993).

5 Seshadri S. et al., 'Plasma homocysteine as a risk factor for dementia and Alzheimer's disease', *New England Journal of Medicine*, 346:476–83 (2002).

6 De Jager C.A., Hogervorst E., Combrinck M., Budge M.M., 'Sensitivity and specificity of neuropsychological tests for mild cognitive impairment, vascular cognitive impairment and Alzheimer's disease', *Psychol Med*, 33(6):1039–50 (Aug 2003).

7 De Jager C.A., Milwain E., Budge M., 'Early detection of isolated memory deficits in the elderly: The need for more sensitive neuropsychological tests', *Psychol Med*, 32(3):483–91 (April 2002).

8 Rowe J.W., Kahn R.L., 'Human aging: usual and successful', *Science*, 237(4811):143–9 (1987); also see the book *Successful Aging* by Kahn and Rowe (Dell: New York, 1998).

9 Smith A.D., 'Homocysteine, B vitamins and cognitive deficit in the elderly', *American Journal of Clinical Nutrition*, 75:785–6 (2002).

10 Bradley K.M. et al., 'Cerebral perfusion SPET correlated with Braak pathological stage in Alzheimer's disease', *Brain*, 125:1772–81 (2002).

11 Jobst K.A. et al., 'Detection in life of confirmed Alzheimer's disease using a simple measurement of medial temporal lobe atrophy by computed tomography', *Lancet*, 340:1179–83 (1992).

12 Jobst K.A. et al., 'Association of atrophy of the medial temporal lobe with reduced blood flow in the posterior parietotemporal cortex in patients with a clinical and pathological diagnosis of Alzheimer's disease', *J Neurol Neurosurg Psychiat*, 55:190–4 (1992).

13 Jobst K.A. et al., 'Rapidly progressing atrophy of medial temporal lobe in Alzheimer's disease', *Lancet*, 343:829–30 (1994).

14 Farris W. et al., 'Insulin-degrading enzyme regulates the levels of insulin, amyloid beta-protein, and the beta-amyloid precursor protein intracellular domain in vivo', *Proc Natl Acad Sci USA*, 100: 4162–7 (2003).

15 Watson G.S. et al., 'The role of insulin resistance in the pathogenesis of Alzheimer's disease: Implications for treatment', *CNS Drugs*, 17:27–45 (2003).

16 Harrell R.F. et al., 'Can nutritional supplements help mentally retarded children? An exploratory study', *Proc Natl Acad Sci*, 78:574–8 (1981).

17 Heininger K., 'A unifying hypothesis of Alzheimer's disease. III Risk factors', *Human Psychopharmacology*, 15:1–70 (2000).

18 Harold D. et al., 'Genome-wide association study identifies variants at CLU and PICALM associated with Alzheimer's disease', *Nature Genetics*, published online 6 September 2009; DOI 10.1038/ng.440.

19 Wilcken B. et al., 'Geographical and ethnic variation in the 677C>T allele of MTHFR', *Journal of Medical Genetics*, 40(8):619–25 (2003).

20 Hoffman A. et al., letter in *Lancet*, 349:151 (1997). Kivipelto M. et al., 'Apolipoprotein E4 magnifies lifestyle risks for dementia: A population-based study', *Journal for Cellular and Molecular Medicine*, 12(6B):2762–71 (2008).

21 Audhya T. et al., Submitted for publication in *Journal of the American Association of Clinical Chemistry*, June 2005.

22 Audhya T. et al., Submitted for publication in *Journal of Nutritional Medicine and Health*.

23 Courtney C. et al., 'Long-term donepezil treatment in 565 patients with Alzheimer's disease (AD2000): Randomised double-blind trial', *Lancet*, 363:2105–15 (2004).

24 Poldinger W. et al., 'A functional-dimensional approach to depression: Serotonin deficiency and target syndrome in a comparison of 5–hydroxytryptophan and fluvoxamine', *Psychopathology*, 24:53–81 (1991).

25 Deijen J.B. et al., 'Tyrosine improves cognitive performance and reduces blood pressure in cadets', *Brain Research Bulletin*, 48:203–9 (1999).

26 Shiah I.S. and Yatham N., 'GABA function in mood disorders: An update and critical review', *Life Sciences*, 63(15):1289–1303 (1998).
27 Seal E.C. et al., 'A randomized, double-blind, placebo-controlled study of oral vitamin B12 supplementation in older patients with subnormal or borderline serum vitamin B12 concentrations', *Journal of the American Geriatric Society*, 50:146–51 (2002).
28 Clarke R. et al., 'Folate, vitamin B12, and serum total homocysteine levels in confirmed Alzheimer disease', *Archives of Neurology*, 55:1449–55 (1998).
29 Ravaglia G. et al., 'Homocysteine and folate as risk factors for dementia and Alzheimer disease' 1, 2, 3 *Am J Clin Nutr*, 82(3):636–43 (2005).
30 Tucker K.L. et al., 'High homocysteine and low B vitamins predict cognitive decline in aging men: the Veterans Affairs Normative Aging Study', *Am J Clin Nutr*, 82(3): 627–35 (2005).
31 Smith A.D., 'The worldwide challenge of the dementias: a role for B vitamins and homocysteine?', *Food Nutr Bull*, 29(2 Suppl):S143–72 (2008).
32 Hogervorst E. et al., 'Plasma homocysteine levels, cerebrovascular risk factors, and cerebral white matter changes (leukoaraiosis) in patients with Alzheimer disease', *Archives of Neurology*, 59:787–93 (2002).
33 Williams J.H. et al., 'Minimal hippocampal width relates to plasma homocysteine in community-dwelling older people', *Age and Ageing*, 31:440–4 (2002).
34 McCaddon A. et al., 'Alzheimer's disease and total plasma aminothiols', *Biol Psychiatry*, 53:254–60 (2003).
35 Miller J.W. et al., 'Homocysteine, vitamin B6, and vascular disease in AD patients', *Neurology*, 58:1471–5 (2002).
36 Esiri M. et al., 'Cerebrovascular disease and threshold for dementia in the early stages of Alzheimer's disease', *Lancet*, 354:919–20 (1999).
37 Seshadri S. et al., 'Plasma homocysteine as a risk factor for dementia and Alzheimer's disease', *New England Journal of Medicine*, 346(7):466–8 (2002).
38 Sachdev P.S. et al., 'Relationship between plasma homocysteine levels and brain atrophy in healthy elderly individuals', *Neurology*, 58:1539–41 (2002).
39 den Heijer T., 'Homocysteine and brain atrophy on MRI of non-demented elderly', *Brain*, 126:170–5 (2003).
40 Wang H.X. et al., 'Vitamin B(12) and folate in relation to the development of Alzheimer's disease', *Neurology*, 56(9):1188–94 (2001).
41 Duthie S.J. et al., 'Homocysteine, B vitamin status, and cognitive function in the elderly', *American Journal of Clinical Nutrition*, 75(5):908–13 (2002).
42 Kado D. et al., 'Homocysteine levels and decline in physical function', *American Journal of Medicine*, 113(7):537–42 (2002).
43 Matsui T. et al., 'Elevated plasma homocysteine levels and risk of silent brain infarction in elderly people', *Stroke*, 32:1116 (2001).

44 Lipton S.A. et al., 'Neurotoxicity associated with dual actions of homocysteine at the N-methyl-D-aspartate receptor', *Proc Natl Acad Sci USA*, 94:5923–8 (1997).
45 Beal M.F. et al., 'Neurochemical characterization of excitotoxin lesions in the cerebral cortex', *J Neuroscience*, 11:147–58 (1991).
46 Clarke R. et al.,'Folate, vitamin B12 and serum total homocysteine levels in confirmed Alzheimer disease', *Arch Neurol*, 55(11):1449–55 (1998).
47 Botteglieri T. et al., 'Plasma total homocysteine levels and the C677T mutation in the methylenetetrahydrofolate reductase (MTHFR) gene: A study in an Italian population with dementia', *Mechanical Ageing Development*, 122(16):2013–23 (2001).
48 Snowdon D.A. et al., 'Serum folate and the severity of atrophy of the neocortex in Alzheimer disease: Findings from the Nun Study', *American Journal of Clinical Nutrition*, 71(4):993–8 (2000).
49 Eto K. et al., 'Brain hydrogen sulfide is severely decreased in Alzheimer's disease', *Biochemical and Biophysical Research Communications*, 293:1485–8 (2002).
50 Sontag E. et al., 'Protein phosphatase 2A methyltransferase links homocysteine metabolism with tau and amyloid precursor protein regulation', *Journal of Neuroscience*, 27(11):2751–9 (2007).
51 McCaddon A. and Kelly C.L., 'Familial Alzheimer's disease and vitamin B12 deficiency', *Age and Ageing*, 23(4):334–7 (1994).
52 McCaddon A. and Kelly C., 'Alzheimer's disease: A "cobalaminergic" hypothesis', *Medical Hypotheses*, 37(3):161–5 (1992).
53 McCaddon A. et al., 'Total serum homocysteine in senile dementia of Alzheimer's type', *International Journal of Geriatric Psychiatry*, 13:235–9 (1998).
54 McCaddon A. et al., 'Homocysteine and cognitive decline in healthy elderly', *Dementia and Geriatric Cognitive Disorders*, 12(5):309–13 (2001).
55 McCaddon A. et al., 'Analogues, ageing and aberrant assimilation of vitamin B12 in Alzheimer's disease, dementia and geriatric cognitive disorders', *Dementia and Geriatric Cognitive Disorders*, 12(2):133–7 (2001).
56 Herbert V. and Herzlich B., 'A proposed model of sequential stages in the development of vitamin B12 deficiency', *Blood*, 66 (suppl 1):45a (1985).
57 McCaddon A. et al., 'Total serum homocysteine in senile dementia of Alzheimer's type', *International Journal of Geriatric Psychiatry*, 13:235–9 (1998).
58 McCaddon A. et al., 'Functional vitamin B12 deficiency and Alzheimer disease', *Neurology*, 58:1395–9 (2002).
59 Aisen P. et al., 'High-dose B vitamin supplementation and cognitive decline in Alzheimer disease', *JAMA*, 300(15):1774–83 (2008).
60 Smith, A.D. et al., 'Homocysteine-lowering by B vitamins slows the rate of accelerated brain atrophy in mild cognitive impairment: a randomized controlled trial', *Public Library of Science ONE*, 5(9) (2010); also see de

Jager C. A. et al., 'B vitamin treatment in mild cognitive impairment', *Public Library of Science ONE* (2011). Douaud, G., et al., 'Preventing Alzheimer's disease-related gray matter atrophy by B-vitamin treatment', *Proc Natl Acad Sci USA* (2013). [Epub ahead of print].

61 Vogiatzoglou A. et al., 'Vitamin B12 status and rate of brain volume loss in community-dwelling elderly', *Neurology*, 71(11):826–32 (2008).

62 Smith A.D. and Refsum H., 'Vitamin B-12 and cognition in the elderly', *Am J Clin Nutr*, 89(2):707S–11S (2009).

63 Tangney C. et al., 'Biochemical indicators of vitamin B12 and folate insufficiency and cognitive decline', *Neurology*, 72(4):361–7 (2009).

64 Vogiatzoglou A. and Smith A.D., 'Dietary sources of vitamin B-12 and their association with plasma vitamin B-12 concentrations in the general population: the Hordaland Homocysteine Study', *American Journal of Clinical Nutrition*, 89(4):1078–87 (2009).

65 Euseen S.J. et al., 'Oral cyanocobalamin supplementation in older people with vitamin B12 deficiency', *Arch Intern Med*, 165(10):1167–72 (2005).

66 Luchsinger J.A. et al., 'Relation of higher folate intake to lower risk of Alzheimer disease in the elderly', *Arch Neurol*, 64(1):86–92 (2007).

67 Durga J. et al., 'Effect of 3–year folic acid supplementation on cognitive function in older adults in the FACIT trial: a randomised, double blind, controlled trial', *Lancet*, 369(9557):208–16 (2007).

68 Morris S.M. et al., 'Folate and vitamin B12 status in relation to anemia, macrocytosis, and cognitive impairment in older Americans in the age of folic acid fortification', *American Journal of Clinical Nutrition*, 85:193–200 (2007).

69 Clarke R. et al., 'Folate, vitamin B12, and serum total homocysteine levels in confirmed Alzheimer disease', *Arch Neurol*, 55(11):1449–55 (1998).

70 Refsum H., 'Low vitamin B-12 status in confirmed Alzheimer's disease as revealed by serum holotranscobalamin', *Journal of Neurology Neurosurgery and Psychiatry*, 74:959–61 (2003).

71 Clarke R. et al., 'Folate, vitamin B12, and serum total homocysteine levels in confirmed Alzheimer disease', *Arch Neurol*, 55(11):1449–55 (1998). See also Oulhaj A. et al., 'Homocysteine as a predictor of cognitive decline in Alzheimer's disease', *Int J Geriatr Psychiatry*, 25(1):82–90 (2010).

72 Koyama K. et al., 'Efficacy of methylcobalamin on lowering total homocysteine plasma concentrations in haemodialysis patients receiving high-dose folate supplementation', *Nephrology Dialysis Transplantation*, 17:916–22 (2002).

73 McGregor D.O. et al., 'Betaine supplementation decreases post-methionine hyperhomocysteinemia in chronic renal failure', *Kidney International*, 61(3):1040–6 (2002).

74 Wassertheil-Smoller S. et al., 'Ostreogen plus progestin increased risk for stroke and probable dementia in postmenopausal women', *Evidence Based Medicine*, 8:170–1 (2003).

75 Perrig W.J. et al., 'The relation between antioxidants and memory performance in the old and very old', *J Am Geriatr Soc*, 45(6):718–24 (1997).

76 Perkins A.J. et al., 'Association of antioxidants with memory in a multiethnic elderly sample using the Third National Health and Nutrition Examination Survey', *Am J Epidemiol*, 150(1):37–44 (1999).

77 Miller J.W., 'Vitamin E and memory: is it vascular protection?', *Nutr Rev*, 58(4):109–11 (2000).

78 Sano M. et al., 'A controlled trial of selegiline, alpha tocopherol or both as treatment of Alzheimer's disease', *New Eng J Med*, 336:1216–22 (1997).

79 Morris M. et al., 'Vitamin E and vitamin C supplement use and risk incident Alzheimer disease', *Alzheimer Dis and Assoc Disorders*, 12:121–6 (1998).

80 Petersen C. et al., 'Vitamin E and donepezil for the treatment of mild cognitive impairment', *New England Journal of Medicine*, 352(23):2379–88 (2005).

81 Cornell U., 9th International Conference on Alzheimer's and Parkinson's Diseases (ADPD) 'Disease with cholinesterase inhibition combined with antioxidants', Abstract 1.

82 Fotuhi M. et al., 'Better cognitive performance in elderly taking antioxidant vitamins E and C supplements in combination with nonsteroidal anti-inflammatory drugs: the Cache County Study', *Alzheimers Dement*, 4(3):223–7 (2008).

83 Morris M. et al., 'Dietary intake of antioxidant nutrients and the risk of incident Alzheimer disease in a biracial community study', *JAMA*, 287(24):3230–7 (2002).

84 Engelhart M. et al., 'Dietary intake of antioxidants and risk of Alzheimer disease', *JAMA*, 287(24):3223–9 (2002).

85 Zandi P. et al., 'Reduced risk of Alzheimer disease in users of antioxidant vitamin supplements: The Cache County Study', *Archives of Neurology*, 61:82–8 (2004).

86 Heart Protection Study Collaborative Group, 'MRC/BHF Heart Protection Study of antioxidant vitamin supplementation in 20,536 high risk individuals', *Lancet*, 360:23–33 (2002).

87 Barberger-Gateau P. et al., 'Dietary patterns and risk of dementia: the Three-city Cohort Study', *Neurology*, 69(20):1921–30 (2007).

88 Mingetti L. et al., 'Peripheral reductive capacity is associated with cognitive performance and survival in Alzheimer's disease', *Journal of Neuroinflammation*, 3:4 (2006).

89 Scarmeas N. et al., 'Mediterranean diet and risk for Alzheimer's disease', *Ann Neurol*, 59(6):912–21 (2006).

90 Nurk E. et al., 'Intake of flavonoid-rich wine, tea, and chocolate by elderly men and women is associated with better cognitive test performance', *J Nutr*, 139(1):120–7 (2009); see also Nurk et al., 'Cognitive performance among the elderly in relation to the intake of 4 plant foods. The Hordaland Health Study', *Br J Nutr* 2010 (in press).

91 Vingtdeux V. et al., 'Therapeutic potential of resveratrol in Alzheimer's disease', *BMC Neurosci*, 9 Suppl 2:S6 (2008).

92 Karuppagounder S.S. et al., 'Dietary supplementation with resveratrol reduces plaque pathology in a transgenic model of Alzheimer's disease', *Neurochem Int*, 54(2):111–18 (2009).

93 Scheltens P. et al., 'Efficacy of a medical food in mild Alzheimer's disease: A randomized, controlled trial', *Alzheimer's & Dementia*, 6(1):1–10 (2010).

94 Bell I.R. et al., 'Brief communication: Vitamin B1, B2, and B6 augmentation of tricyclic antidepressant treatment in geriatric depression with cognitive dysfunction', *Journal of the American College of Nutrition*, 11(2):159–63 (1992).

95 Morris M. et al., 'Dietary niacin and the risk of incident Alzheimer's disease and of cognitive decline', *Journal of Neurology Neurosurgery and Psychiatry*, 75:1093–9 (2004).

96 Brooks J.O. et al., 'Acetyl-L-carnitine slows decline in younger patients with Alzheimer's disease: A reanalysis of a double-blind, placebo-controlled study using the trilinear approach', *Int Psychogeriatr*, 10:193–203 (1998).

97 Bruno G. et al., 'Acetyl-L-carnitine in Alzheimer disease: A short-term study on CSF neurotransmitters and neuropeptides', *Alzheimer Dis Assoc Disord*, 9:128–31 (1995).

98 Salvioli G., Neri M., 'L-acetylcarnitine treatment of mental decline in the elderly', *Drugs Exp Clin Res*, 20:169–76 (1994).

99 Jiankang Liu et al., 'Memory loss in old rats is associated with brain mitochondrial decay and RNA/DNA oxidation: Partial reversal by feeding acetyl-L-carnitine and/or R-lipoic acid', *Proc Natl Acad Sci*, 99:2356–61 (2002).

100 Hagen T.M. et al., 'Feeding acetyl-L-carnitine and lipoic acid to old rats significantly improves metabolic function while decreasing oxidative stress', *Proc Natl Acad Sci*, 99:1870–5 (2002).

101 Jiankang Liu et al., 'Age-associated mitochondrial oxidative decay: Improvement of carnitine acetyltransferase substrate-binding affinity and activity in brain by feeding old rats acetyl-L-carnitine and/or R-lipoic acid', *Proc Natl Acad Sci*, 99:1876–81 (2002).

102 Jing H. et al., 'Effects of glutamate and glutamine on learning and memory of rats', *Wei Sheng Yan Jiu*, 29:40–2 (2000).

103 Leventhal A.G. et al., 'GABA and its agonists improved visual cortical function in senescent monkeys', *Science*, 300:812–15 (2003).

104 Morris M. et al., 'Consumption of fish and n-3 fatty acids and risk of incident Alzheimer disease', *Archives of Neurology*, 60:940–6 (2003).

105 Barberger-Gateau P. et al., 'Dietary patterns and risk of dementia: the Three-city Cohort Study', *Neurology*, 69(20):1921–30 (2007).

106 Calon F. et al., 'Docosahexaenoic acid protects from dendritic pathology in an Alzheimer's disease mouse model', *Neuron*, 43:633–45 (2004).

107 Chiu C.C. et al., 'The effects of omega-3 fatty acids monotherapy in Alzheimer's disease and mild cognitive impairment: a preliminary randomized double-blind placebo-controlled study', *Progress in Neuro-Psychopharmacology and Biological Psychiatry*, 32(6):1538–44 (2008).

108 Kalmijn S. et al., 'Dietary fat intake and the risk of incident dementia in the Rotterdam Study', *Ann Neurol*, 42(5):776–82 (1997); Engelhart M.J. et al., 'Diet and risk of dementia: Does fat matter?: the Rotterdam Study', *Neurology*, 59(12):1915–21 (2002); Morris M.C. et al., 'Consumption of fish and n-3 fatty acids and risk of incident Alzheimer disease', *Arch Neurol*, 60(7):940–6 (2003).

109 Hypponen E. et al., 'Hypovitaminosis D in British adults at age 45 y: nationwide cohort study of dietary and lifestyle predictors', *Am J Clin Nutr*, 85(3):860–8 (2007).

110 Llewellyn D.J. et al., 'Serum 25–hydroxyvitamin D concentration and cognitive impairment', *J Geriatr Psychiatry Neurol*, 22(3):188–95 (2009).

111 Annweiler C. et al., 'Low serum vitamin D concentrations in Alzheimer's disease: a systematic review and meta-analysis', *J Alzheimer's Dis*, 33(3):659–74 (2013).

112 Lu'o'ng K.V., Nguyen L.T., 'The role of vitamin D in Alzheimer's disease: possible genetic and cell signaling mechanisms', *Am J Alzheimer's Dis Other Demen*, 28(2):126–36 (2013).

113 Pyapali G. et al., 'Prenatal dietary choline supplementation', *Journal of Neurophysiology*, 79(4):1790–6 (1998); and Meck W.H. et al., 'Characterization of the facilitative effects of perinatal choline supplementation on timing and temporal memory', *Neuroreport*, 8(13):2831–5 (1997).

114 Chung S.Y. et al., 'Administration of phosphatidylcholine increases brain acetylcholine concentration and improves memory in mice with dementia', *J Nutr*, 125(6):1484–9 (1995).

115 Wurtman R.J. and Zeisel S.H., 'Brain choline: its sources and effects on the synthesis and release of acetylcholine', *Aging*, 19:303–13 (1992).

116 Cansev M. et al., 'Oral administration of circulating precursors for membrane phosphatides can promote the synthesis of new brain synapses', *Alzheimers Dement*, 4(1 Suppl 1):S153–68 (2008).

117 De Jesus Moreno Moreno M., 'Cognitive improvement in mild to moderate Alzheimer's dementia after treatment with the acetylcholine precursor choline alfoscerate: a multicenter, double-blind, randomized, placebo-controlled trial', *Clin Ther*, 25(1):178–93 (2003).

118 McDaniel M.A. et al., '"Brain-specific" nutrients: A memory cure?', *Nutrition*, 19:957–75 (2003).

119 Ladd S.L., Sommer S.A., LaBerge S., Toscano W., 'Effect of phosphatidylcholine on explicit memory', *Clin Neuropharmacol*, 16(6):540–9 (1993).

120 Canty D.J. and Zeisel S.H., 'Lecithin and choline in human health and disease', *Nutr Rev*, 52(10):327–39 (1994).

121 Amenta F. et al., 'The cholinergic approach for the treatment of vascular dementia: Evidence from pre-clinical and clinical studies', *Clin Exp Hypertens*, 24(7–8):697–713 (Oct–Nov 2002).

122 Dimpfel W. et al., 'Source density analysis of functional topographical EEG: Monitoring of cognitive drug action', *European Journal of Medical Research*, 1(6):283–90 (1996).

123 Cases published in Dean W., Morgenthaler J. and Fowkes S., *Smart Drugs II: The Next Generation*, ISBN 0 9627 4187 6, Smart Publications, 1993, reproduced with their kind permission.

124 Chung S.Y. et al., 'Administration of phosphatidylcholine increases brain acetylcholine concentration and improves memory in mice with dementia', *J Nutr*, 125: 1484–9 (1995).

125 Ferris S.H. et al., 'Senile dementia: Treatment with Deanol', *J Am Geriatr Soc*, 25:241–4 (1977).

126 Crook T. et al., 'Effects of phosphatidyl serine in age-associated memory impairment', *Neurology*, 41(5):644–9 (1991).

127 Suzuki S. et al., 'Oral administration of soybean lecithin transphosphatidylated phosphatidylserine improves memory impairment in aged rats', *J Nutr*, 131:2951–6 (2001).

128 Crook T. et al., 'Effects of phosphatidyl serine in age-associated memory impairment', *Neurology*, 41(5):644–9 (1991).

129 Gindin J. et al., 'The effect of plant phosphatidylserine on age-associated memory impairment and mood in the functioning elderly', *Geriatric Inst for Ed Res*, and Dept of Geriatrics, Kaplan Hospital, Rhovot, Israel (1995).

130 Maggioni M. et al., 'Effects of phosphatidylserine therapy in geriatric subjects with depressive disorders', *Acta Psychiatr Scand*, 81:265–70 (1990).

131 Reported at the International Congress of Nutrition in Kyoto, Japan, by Dr R. Alfin-Slater (1975).

132 Saxton J. et al., 'Alcohol, dementia, and Alzheimer's disease: Comparison of neuropsychological profiles', *J Geriatr Psychiatry Neurol*, 13:141–9 (2000).

133 den Heijer T. et al., 'Alcohol intake in relation to brain magnetic resonance imaging findings in older persons without dementia', *Am J Clin Nutr*, 80:992–7 (2004).

134 Edwin D. et al., 'Cognitive impairment in alcoholic and nonalcoholic cirrhotic patients', *Hepatology*, 30:1363–7 (1999).

135 Bleich S. et al., 'Moderate alcohol consumption in social drinkers raises plasma homocysteine levels: A contradiction to the "French Paradox"?', *Alcohol*, 36:189–92 (2000).
136 van der Gaag M.S. et al., 'Effect of consumption of red wine, spirits, and beer on serum homocysteine', *Lancet*, 355:1522 (2000).
137 Mayer O. et al., 'A population study of the influence of beer consumption on folate and homocysteine concentrations', *Eur J Clin Nutr*, 55:605–9 (2001).
138 Dixon J.B. et al., 'Reduced plasma homocysteine in obese red wine consumers: A potential contributor to reduced cardiovascular risk status', *Eur J Clin Nutr*, 56:608–14 (2002).
139 Luchsinger J.A. et al., 'Hyperinsulinemia and risk of Alzheimer disease', *Neurology*, 63:1187–92 (2004).
140 Abbatecola A.M. et al., 'Insulin resistance and executive dysfunction in older persons', *J Am Geriatr Soc*, 52:1713–18 (2004).
141 Xu W.L. et al., 'Diabetes mellitus and risk of dementia in the Kungsholmen project: A 6–year follow-up study', *Neurology*, 63:1181–6 (2004).
142 Hassing L.B. et al., 'Type 2 diabetes mellitus contributes to cognitive decline in old age: A longitudinal population-based study', *J Int Neuropsychol Soc*, 10:599–607 (2004).
143 Yaffe K. et al., 'Diabetes, impaired fasting glucose, and development of cognitive impairment in older women', *Neurology*, 63:658–63 (2004).
144 Arvanitakis Z. et al., 'Diabetes mellitus and risk of Alzheimer's disease and decline in cognitive function', *Arch Neurol*, 61:661–6 (2004).
145 Yaffe K. et al., 'Glycosylated hemoglobin level and development of mild cognitive impairment or dementia in older women', *J Nutr Health Aging*, 10(4):293–5 (2006).
146 Cleary J. et al., 'Naloxone effects of sugar-motivated behaviour', *Psychopharmacology*, 176:110–14 (1996).
147 Czirr S.A. and Reid L.D., 'Demonstrating morphine's potentiating effects on sucrose intake', *Brain Research Bulletin*, 17:639–42 (1986).
148 Blass E. et al., 'Interactions between sucrose, pain, isolation distress', *Pharmacology, Biochemistry of Behaviour*, 26:483–9 (1986).
149 Leventhal L. et al., 'Selective actions of central mu and kappa opioid antagonists upon sucrose intake in sham-fed rats', *Brain Research*, 685:205–10 (1995).
150 Moles A. and Cooper S., 'Opioid modulation of sucrose intake in CD-1 mice', *Physiology and Behaviour*, 58:791–6 (1995).
151 Cheraskin E. and Ringsdorf W.M., 'A biochemical denominator in the primary prevention of alcoholism', *Journal of Orthomolecular Psychiatry*, 9(3):158–63 (1980).
152 Pert C.B., *The Molecules of Emotion* (London: Pocket Books, 1999).

153 Wurtman R. and Wurtman J., 'Carbohydrates and depression', *Scientific American*, 260:68–75 (1989).

154 Sapolsky R.M., 'Why stress is bad for your brain', *Science*, 273:749–50 (1995).

155 Bremner J.D. et al., 'MRI-based measurement of hippocampal volume in patients with combat-related posttraumatic stress disorder', *Am J Psychiatry*, 152:973–81 (1995).

156 Kirschbaum C. et al., 'Stress- and treatment-induced elevations of cortisol levels associated with impaired declarative memory in healthy adults', *Life Sci*, 58(17):1475–83 (1996).

157 Newcomer J.W. et al., 'Decreased memory performance in healthy humans induced by stress-level cortisol treatment', *Arch Gen Psychiatry*, 56:527–33 (1999).

158 Giubilei F. et al., 'Altered circadian cortisol secretion in Alzheimer's disease: clinical and neuroradiological aspects', *J Neurosci Res*, 66:262–5 (2001).

159 Crapper McLachlan D.R. et al., 'Intramuscular desferrioxamine in patients with Alzheimer's disease', *Lancet*, 337:1304–8 (1991).

160 Polizzi S. et al., 'Neurotoxic effects of aluminium among foundry workers and Alzheimer's disease', *Neurotoxicology*, 23:761–74 (2002).

161 Rifat S.L. et al., 'Effect of exposure of miners to aluminium powder', *Lancet*, 336:1162–5 (1990).

162 Suay Llopis L. et al., 'Review of studies on exposure to aluminum and Alzheimer's disease', *Rev Esp Salud Publica*, 76:645–58 (2002).

163 Campbell A., 'The potential role of aluminium in Alzheimer's disease', *Nephrology Dialysis Transplantation*, 17:17–20 (2002).

164 Landsberg J.P. et al., 'Absence of aluminium in neuritic plaque cores in Alzheimer's disease', *Nature*, 360:65–8 (1992).

165 Makjanic J. et al., 'Absence of aluminium in neurofibrillary tangles in Alzheimer's disease', *Neurosci Lett*, 240:123–6 (1998).

166 Beauchemin D. and Kisilevsky R., 'A method based on ICP-MS for the analysis of Alzheimer's amyloid plaques', *Anal Chem*, 70:1026–9 (1998).

167 Wenstrup D. et al., 'Trace element imbalances in isolated subcellular fractions of Alzheimer's disease patients', *Brain Research*, 553:125–31 (1990).

168 Hock C. et al., 'Increased blood mercury levels in patients with Alzheimer's disease', *J Neural Transm*, 105:59–68 (1998).

169 Leong C.C. et al., 'Retrograde degeneration of neurite membrane structural integrity of nerve growth cones following in vitro exposure to mercury', *Neuroreport*, 12:733–7 (2001). See also www.commons.ucalgary. ca/mercury.

170 Pendergrass J.C. et al., 'Mercury vapor inhalation inhibits binding of GTP to tubulin in rat brain: Similarity to a molecular lesion in Alzheimer's disease brain', *Neurotoxicology*, 18:315–24 (1997).

171 Schuurs A.H., de Wolff F.A., 'Relation between mercury and Alzheimer's disease?' *Ned Tijdschr Tandheelkd*, 104(6):219–22 (1997) (in Dutch).

172 Cornett, C.R. et al., 'Trace elements in Alzheimer's disease pituitary glands', *Biol Trace Elem Res*, 62:107–14 (1998).
173 Saxe S.R. et al., 'Alzheimer's disease, dental amalgam and mercury', *J Am Dent Assoc*, 130:191–9 (1999).
174 Carta P. et al., 'Sub-clinical neurobehavioral abnormalities associated with low level of mercury exposure through fish consumption', *Neurotoxicology*, 24:617–23 (2003).
175 Dorea J. et al., 'Mercury in hair and in fish consumed by Riparian women of the Rio Negro, Amazon, Brazil', *Int J Environ Health Res*, 13(3):239–48 (2003).
176 Ritchie C.W. et al., 'Metal-protein attenuation with iodochlorhydroxyquin (clioquinol) targeting Abeta amyloid deposition and toxicity in Alzheimer disease: A pilot phase 2 clinical trial', *Arch Neurol*, 60:1685–91 (2003).
177 Morris M.C. et al., 'Dietary copper and high saturated and trans fat intakes associated with cognitive decline', *Arch Neurol*, 63(8):1085–8 (2006).
178 Constantinidis J., 'Hypothesis regarding amyloid and zinc in the pathogenesis of Alzheimer disease: Potential for preventive intervention', *Alzheimer Dis Assoc Disord*, 5:31–5 (1991).
179 Kleijnin J. and Knipschild P., 'Ginkgo biloba', *Lancet*, 340:1136–9 (1992).
180 Le Bars P.L., 'A placebo-controlled, double-blind, randomised trial on an extract of Ginkgo biloba for dementia', *JAMA*, 278(16):1327–32 (1997).
181 Birks J., 'Ginkgo biloba for cognitive impairment and dementia', *Cochrane Database Syst Rev*, (4): CD003120 (2002).
182 van Dongen M. et al., 'Ginkgo for elderly people with dementia and age-associated memory impairment: A randomized clinical trial', *J Clin Epidemiol*, 56:367–76 (2003).
183 Solomon P.R. et al., 'Ginkgo for memory enhancement: A randomized controlled trial', *JAMA*, 288:835–40 (2002).
184 Mix J.A. and Crews W.D., 'A double-blind, placebo-controlled, randomized trial of Ginkgo biloba extract EGb 761 in a sample of cognitively intact older adults: Neuropsychological findings', *Hum Psychopharmacol*, 17(6):267–77 (Aug 2002).
185 Birks J. and Grimley Evans J. 'Ginkgo biloba for cognitive impairment and dementia', *Cochrane Database Syst Rev*, (2):CD003120 (2007).
186 Huguet F. et al., 'Decreased cerebral 5–HT1A receptors during aging: Reversal by Ginkgo biloba extract', *J Pharm Pharmacol*, 46:316–18 (1994).
187 Cohen A.J. and Bartlik B., 'Ginkgo biloba for antidepressant-induced sexual dysfunction', *J Sex Marital Thera*, 124(2):139–43 (1998).
188 Spinella M., *The Psychopharmacology of Herbal Medicine*, MIT Press (2001).
189 Hindmarch I. et al., 'Efficacy and tolerance of vinpocetine in ambulant patients suffering from mild to moderate organic psychosyndromes', *Int Clin Psychopharmacol*, 6:31–43 (1991).

190 Balestreri R. et al., 'A double-blind placebo controlled evaluation of the safety and efficacy of vinpocetine in the treatment of patients with chronic vascular senile cerebral dysfunction', *J Am Geriatr Soc*, 35:425–30 (1987).

191 Subhan Z. and Hindmarch I., 'Psychopharmacological effects of vinpocetine in normal healthy volunteers', *Eur J Clin Pharmacol*, 28:567–71 (1985).

192 Szatmari S.Z. and Whitehouse P.J., 'Vinpocetine for cognitive impairment and dementia', *Cochrane Database Syst Rev*, (1):CD003119 (2003).

193 Scholey A.B. et al., 'Acute, dose-dependent cognitive effects of Ginkgo biloba, Panax ginseng and their combination in healthy young volunteers: Differential interactions with cognitive demand', *Hum Psychopharmacol*, 17:35–44 (2002).

194 Kennedy D.O. et al., 'Ginseng: Potential for the enhancement of cognitive performance and mood', *Pharmacol Biochem Behav*, 75:687–700 (2003).

195 Yang F. et al., 'Curcumin inhibits formation of amyloid beta oligomers and fibrils, binds plaques, and reduces amyloid in vivo', *J Biol Chem*, 280(7):5892–901 (2005).

196 Zangara A., 'The psychopharmacology of huperzine A: An alkaloid with cognitive enhancing and neuroprotective properties of interest in the treatment of Alzheimer's disease', *Pharmacol Biochem Behav*, 75:675–86 (2003).

197 Gu Y. et al., 'Food combination and Alzheimer Disease Risk', *Archives of Neurology*, 67(6) (2010).

198 Colcombe S.J. et al., 'Neurocognitive aging and cardiovascular fitness: recent findings and future directions', *J Mol Neurosci*, 24:9–14 (2004).

199 Callaghan P., 'Exercise: A neglected intervention in mental health care?', *J Psychiatr Ment Health Nurs*, 11:476–83 (2004).

200 Lytle M.E. et al., 'Exercise level and cognitive decline: the MoVIES project', *Alzheimer Dis Assoc Disord*, 18:57–64 (2004).

201 Sobel B.P., 'Bingo vs physical intervention in stimulating short-term cognition in Alzheimer's disease patients', *Am J Alzheimers Dis Other Demen*, 16:115–20 (2001).

202 Laurin D. et al., 'Physical activity and risk of cognitive impairment and dementia in elderly persons', *Arch Neurol*, 58:498–504 (2001).

203 Wilson R.S. et al., 'Cognitive activity and incident AD in a population-based sample of older persons', *Neurology*, 59:1910–14 (2002).

204 Verghese J. et al., 'Leisure activities and the risk of dementia in the elderly', *The New England Journal of Medicine*, 348:2508–16 (2003).

205 Wilson R.S. et al., 'Participation in cognitively stimulating activities and risk of incident Alzheimer disease', *JAMA*, 287:742–8 (2002).

206 Crawford J.G., 'Alzheimer's disease risk factors as related to cerebral blood flow', *Med Hypotheses*, 46:367–77 (1996).

207 Osawa A. et al., 'Relationship between cognitive function and regional cerebral blood flow in different types of dementia', *Disabil Rehabil*, 26:739–45 (2004).

208 Colcombe S. et al., 'Aerobic exercise training increases brain volume in aging humans', *J Gerontol A Biol Sci Med Sci*, 61(11):1166–70 (2006).

209 Rovio S. et al., 'Leisure-time physical activity at midlife and the risk of dementia and Alzheimer's disease', *Lancet Neurol*, 4(11):705–11 (2005).

210 Laurin D. et al., 'Physical activity and risk of cognitive impairment and dementia in elderly persons', *Arch Neuro*, 58:498–504 (2001).

211 Larson E.B. et al., 'Exercise is associated with reduced risk for incident dementia among persons 65 years of age and older', *Ann Intern Med*, 144(2):73–81 (2006).

212 Satoh T. et al., 'Walking exercise and improved neuropsychological functioning in elderly patients with cardiac disease', *J Intern Med*, 238:423–8 (1995).

213 Ravaglia G. et al., 'Physical activity and dementia risk in the elderly: findings from a prospective Italian study', *Neurology*, 70:1786–94 (2008).

214 Lautenschlager N. et al., 'Effect of physical activity on cognitive function in older adults at risk for Alzheimer disease: a randomized trial', *JAMA*, 300(9):1027–37 (2008).

215 Colcombe S.J. et al., 'Aerobic fitness reduces brain tissue loss in aging humans', *J Gerontol A Biol Sci Med Sci*, 58:176–80 (2003).

216 Teri L. et al., 'Exercise plus behavioral management in patients with Alzheimer disease: A randomized controlled trial', *JAMA*, 290:2015–22 (2003).

217 Gustafson D. et al., 'An 18–year follow-up of overweight and risk of Alzheimer disease', *Arch Intern Med*, 14;163(13):1524–8 (July 2003).

218 Naveen K.V. et al., 'Yoga breathing through a particular nostril increases spatial memory scores without lateralized effects', *Psychol Rep*, 81:555–61 (1997).

219 Jella S.A. et al., 'The effects of unilateral forced nostril breathing on cognitive performance', *Int J Neurosci*, 73:61–8 (1993).

220 Graf A. et al., 'The effects of light therapy on mini-mental state examination scores in demented patients', *Biol Psychiatry*, 50:725–7 (2001).

221 Gray R. et al., 'Long-term donepezil treatment in 565 patients with Alzheimer's disease (AD2000): Randomised double-blind trial', *Lancet*, 363:2105–15 (2004).

222 Knoll research reported in Dean W. et al., *Smart Drugs II: The next generation*, ISBN 0 9627 4187 6, Smart Publications (1993).

223 Khalsa D.S., 'Integrated medicine and the prevention and reversal of memory loss', *Alternative Therapies in Health and Medicine*, 4(6):38–43 (1998); and Wu R.M. et al., 'Suppression of hydroxyl radical formation and

protection of nigral neurons by l-deprenyl (segeliline)', *Annals of the New York Academy of Sciences*, 786:379–90 (1996).

224 Bartus R.T. et al.,'Profound effects of combining choline and piracetam on memory enhancement', *Neurobiology of Ageing*, 2:105–11 (1981).

225 Elsworth J.D. et al., 'Deprenyl administration in man: A selective MAO-B inhibitor without the "cheese effect"', *Psychopharmacology (Berl)*, 57(1):33–8 (1978).

226 Ward D. and Morgenthaler J., *Smart Drugs and Nutrients*, Smart Publications, (1990), pp. 42–3.

227 Tariska P. and Paksy A., 'Cognitive enhancement effect of piracetam in patients with mild cognitive impairment and dementia', *Orv Hetil*, 141(22):1189–93 (2000).

228 Mindus P. et al.,'Piracetam-induced improvement of mental performance: A controlled study on normally aging individuals', *Acta Psychiat Scand*, 54:150–60 (1976).

229 Israel L. et al., 'Drug therapy and memory training programs: A double-blind randomized trial of general practice patients with age-associated memory impairment', *Int Psychogeriatr*, 6(2):155–70 (1994).

230 Pilch H. and Muller W.E., 'Chronic treatment with piracetam elevates muscarinic cholinergic receptor density in the frontal cortex of aged mice', *Pharmacopsychiatry*, 21(6):324–5 (1988).

231 Schneider L.S. and Olin J.T., 'Overview of clinical trials of hydergine in dementia', *Arch Neurol*, 51(8):787–98 (1994).

232 Ibid.

233 Wassertheil-Smoller S. et al., 'Ostreogen plus progestin increased risk for stroke and probable dementia in postmenopausal women', *Evidence Based Medicine*, 8:170–1 (2003).

Recommended Reading

Braverman, E., *The Edge Effect*, Sterling (2004)

Holford, P., *The Optimum Nutrition Bible*, Piatkus (2009)

Holford, P., *Optimum Nutrition for the Mind*, Piatkus (2010)

Holford, P. and Braly J., *The H Factor*, Piatkus (2007)

Schmidt, M., *Smart Fats*, Frog (1997)

Warren, T., *Beating Alzheimer's*, Avery (1991)

Warren, T., *Reversing Chronic Disease*, Tom Warren (2003)

Useful Addresses

Food for the Brain is an educational charity that promotes the link between optimum nutrition and mental health. Founded by Patrick Holford, it exists to inform the public about the role of nutrition in mental health; to promote the nutrition connection to health professionals, policy makers and sufferers; and to provide resources to encourage more research and implementation of nutritional strategies.

Visit our website for:

- A FREE e-letter on nutritional approaches to mental health
- The latest research on drug-free approaches to mental health
- Mental health seminars and events near you
- Details on the Brain Bio Centre, Britain's only clinic specialising in the optimum nutrition approach to mental health (see page 248).

Visit www.foodforthebrain.org

General mental health/Alzheimer's

Alzheimer's Society This is the UK's leading care and research charity for people with dementia, their families and carers. While they are not particularly progressive on nutritional approaches, they provide plenty of information about all forms of dementia. They also have local support groups. Visit www.alzheimers.org.uk; contact them at Alzheimer's Society, Gordon House, 10 Greencoat Place, London SW1P 1PH; or telephone 020 7306 0606.

Cognitive Enhancement Research Institute (CERI) gives up-to-date information on mind and memory boosters. This website has many interesting features, and international listings for suppliers of smart drugs and nutrients, and will keep you updated on topical issues. Visit www.ceri.com. For books and products, also visit www.smart-publications.com.

International Society for Orthomolecular Medicine Orthomolecular medicine is the practice of preventing and treating disease by providing the body with optimal amounts of substances which are natural to the body. The Society's purpose is to further the advancement of orthomolecular medicine throughout the world. You can find details of practitioners of this approach around the world from their website www.orthomed.org/isom/isom.htm. Also visit their website www.orthomed.org for further information on this approach.

Mental Health Foundation is an organisation that provides all sorts of useful information on mental health, although nothing specifically on nutrition. They have a very comprehensive list of mental health organisations. Visit www.mentalhealth.org.uk; telephone their helpline on 020 7802 0302; or contact their UK office at 7th Floor, 83 Victoria Street, London SW1H 0HW.

Safe Harbor Project, based in the US, collects and distributes information on non-pharmaceutical approaches to mental disorders via their website, www.alternativementalhealth.com, which is full of useful information and articles. Here you can subscribe to their free e-newsletter, Alternative Mental Health News, which is also kindly available at www.mentalhealthproject.com, via the UK-based Mental Health Project.

Nutritional treatment and nutrition practitioners

The Brain Bio Centre is a London-based treatment centre, set up by the Mental Health Project, putting the optimum nutrition approach into practice for those with mental health problems, including Alzheimer's, dementia, memory loss, depression, anxiety, learning difficulties, dyslexia, ADHD, autism and schizophrenia. For details and to order an Information Pack, visit www.mentalhealthproject.com or telephone 020 332 9600.

The Institute for Optimum Nutrition (ION) offers a three-year foundation degree course in nutritional therapy that includes training in the optimum nutrition approach to mental health. There is a clinic, a list of nutrition practitioners across the UK, an information service and a quarterly journal, *Optimum Nutrition.* Visit www.ion.ac.uk. Address: Avalon House, 72 Lower Mortlake Road, Richmond, TW9 2JY. Telephone: 020 8614 7800.

Nutritional therapy and consultations To find a nutritional therapist near you who I recommend, visit www.patrickholford.com. This service gives details on whom to see in the UK as well as internationally. If there is no one available near by, you can always do an on-line assessment – see below.

On-Line 100% Health Programme How 100% healthy are you? Find out with our health check and comprehensive personalised 100% Health Programme giving you a personalised action plan, including diet and supplements. Visit www.patrickholford.com.

Zest4Life is a health and nutrition club, based on low-GL principles, that provides advice, coaching and support for losing weight and gaining health through a series of weekly meetings. For more information, visit www.zest4life.eu.

Laboratory testing

Homocysteine testing is available through YorkTest Laboratories using a home test kit that allows you to take your own pinprick blood sample and return it to the lab for analysis. Visit www.yorktest.com; freephone 0800 0746185 or contact FREEPOST NEA5 243, York YO19 5ZZ. You may also be able to have your homocysteine level tested through your doctor. YorkTest also has a GL Check home test kit which measures your level of glycosylated haemoglobin (also called HbA1C).

Neurotransmitter testing is only available for patients at the Brain Bio Centre (see above).

Hair Mineral Analyses are available from Trace Elements, Inc (US), a leading laboratory for hair mineral analysis for healthcare professionals worldwide. Visit www.traceelements.com for more details or contact the UK agent Mineral Check at 62 Cross Keys, Bearsted, Maidstone, Kent ME14 4HR; telephone 01622 630044 or visit www.mineralcheck.com.

All of the tests are available through the Brain Bio Centre for patients only.

Stress reduction – t'ai chi, yoga and Psychocalisthenics

T'ai chi and qigong The Tai Chi Union for Great Britain provides details of teachers near you, events and news. Visit www.taichiunion.com. Also contact The London School of T'ai Chi Chuan and Traditional Health Resources, visit http://taichi.gn.apc.org/ or telephone 020 8566 1677.

Yoga The British Wheel of Yoga can put you in touch with a yoga school or teacher in your area. Visit www.bwy.org.uk/; telephone 01529 306851 or email office@bwy.org.uk.

Psychocalisthenics is an excellent exercise system that takes less than 20 minutes a day, and develops strength, suppleness and stamina, as well as generating vital energy. The best way to learn it is to do the Psychocalisthenics Training. See www.patrickholford.com (events) for details. Also available is the book *Master Level Exercise: Psychocalisthenics* and the Psychocalisthenics CD and DVD, available from www.patrickholford.com (shop). For further information please see www.pcals.com.

Health products

Sugar alternative – XyloBrit (xylitol) this low-GL natural sugar alternative is available from www.totallynourish.com.

CherryActive is sold in a highly concentrated juice format. Mix a 30ml serving with 250ml water to make a deliciously healthy, low-GL cherry juice drink. Each 946ml bottle contains the juice from over 3,000 cherries – that's half a tree's worth – and contains a month's supply. CherryActive is also available as a dried cherry snack and in capsules. For more information and to order, visit www.totallynourish.com (see page 253).

Water filters There are many water filters on the market. One of the best is offered by The Fresh Water Filter Company, who produce mains-attached water-filtering units using gravity rather than reverse osmosis (which can filter out some useful minerals as well). You can buy a whole-house filter or an under-sink version. Visit www.totallynourish.com or www.freshwaterfilter.com.

Supplements and suppliers

Finding your own perfect supplement programme can be confusing, but my website, www.patrickholford.com, offers useful guidance.

The backbone of a good supplement programme is:

- A high strength multivitamin
- Additional vitamin C
- An essential fat supplement containing omega-3 and omega-6 oils.

In this section are examples of supplements that provide the herbs and nutrients at the levels discussed in this book. The addresses of the companies whose products I've referred to are given at the end.

Supplements

Antioxidants

A good all-round antioxidant complex should provide vitamin A (beta-carotene and/or retinol), vitamins C and E, zinc, selenium, glutathione or cysteine, anthocyanidins of berry extracts, lipoic acid and co-enzyme Q10. Two products that fulfil this criteria are the AGE Antioxidant from the Patrick Holford range or Solgar's Advanced Antioxidant Nutrients. Complexes of bioflavonoids, often found together with vitamin C, are available from both companies.

Brain support and phospholipid supplements

The brain needs essential fats (see below), phospholipids such as phosphatidyl choline and phosphatidyl serine, plus other key nutrients to function optimally. These include pyroglutamate and DMAE, from which the brain can make phosphatidyl choline. Brain Food Formula from the Patrick Holford range contains all these, plus some ginkgo.

Phosphatidyl serine is available in 100mg capsules from a number of companies. Phosphatidyl choline (PC) can be found in lecithin granules. Higher Nature sells a 'high PC' lecithin. Ask in your local health food store.

Essential fats and fish oil supplements

The most important omega-3 fats are DHA and EPA, the richest source being cod liver oil. The most important omega-6 fat is GLA, the richest source being borage (also known as starflower) oil. My favourite supplement is Essential Omegas from the Patrick Holford range, which provides a highly concentrated mix of EPA, DHA and GLA. They also produce a Mega EPA fish oil supplement that is good value, as is Seven Seas Extra High Strength Cod Liver Oil. Both these products have consistently proven the purest when tested for PCB residues, which are in almost all fish. Cod liver oil also contains vitamin A.

Homocysteine/Methyl nutrient complexes

A good methyl nutrient complex should contain at least B6, B12 and folic acid. Some formulas also contain vitamin B2, trimethylglycine (TMG), zinc and N-acetyl cysteine. Three products that fulfil this criteria are Connect from the Patrick Holford range, which contains them all; Solgar's GOLD SPECIFICS Homocysteine Modulators, which contains TMG, vitamin B6, vitamin B12 and folic acid; and Higher Nature's 'H Factors', which contains vitamins B2, B6, B12, folic acid and zinc, plus TMG (see www.highernature.co.uk).

Multivitamin and mineral supplements

Supplementing the right multivitamin is the most important supplement decision you make. Most multis are based on RDA levels of nutrients, which are not the same as optimum nutrition levels. A good multivitamin, based on optimum nutrition levels, is the Optimum Nutrition Formula from the Patrick Holford range. Another is Solgar's VM2000. Both of these recommend taking two tablets a day. The Optimum Nutrition Formula has higher mineral levels, especially for calcium and magnesium. Ideally, take a multivitamin and mineral with an extra 1g of vitamin C.

Smart drugs and nutrients

These can be bought by mail order from abroad and shipped to UK customers for personal use. Search the web for US suppliers, most of whom ship to the UK, or visit www.smart-publications.com/store/index.html. Also see www.ceri.com.

Supplement suppliers

The following companies produce good-quality supplements that are widely available in the UK.

BioCare offers an extensive range of nutritional and herbal supplements. Their products are stocked by most good health-food shops. Visit www.biocare.co.uk or telephone 0121 433 3727. They are also available by mail order from Totally Nourish (www.totallynourish.com).

Patrick Holford's range of daily supplement 'packs' are good for travelling or when you are away from home. Other supplements are socked by most good health-food stores, including Holland & Barrett – see www.hollandandbarrett.com. They are also available by mail order from www.totallynourish.com.

Totally Nourish is an 'e'-health shop that stocks many high quality health products, including home test kits and supplements. Visit www.totallynourish.com or telephone 0800 085 7749 (freephone within the UK).

Solgar products are available in most independent health-food shops. For information, visit www.solgar-vitamins.co.uk or telephone 01442 890355.

And in other regions

South Africa

The original PATRICK HOLFORD vitamin and supplement brand from the UK is now available in South Africa through leading health food shops, Dis-Chem and Clicks leading retail pharmacies. They are also available online direct from www.holforddirect.co.za, by post or by courier direct to your door. PATRICK HOLFORD supplements, books and CDs can also be ordered by phone on 011 2654554.

Australia

Solgar supplements are available in Australia. Visit www.solgar.com.au or telephone 1800 029 871 (free call) for your nearest supplier. Another good brand is Blackmores.

New Zealand

BioCare products (see above) are available in New Zealand through Pacific Health, PO Box 56248, Dominion Road, Auckland 1446, New Zealand, www.pachealth.co.nz or contact 0064 9815 0707.

Singapore

BioCare (see above) and Solgar products are available in Singapore through Essential Living. Visit www.essliv.com or telephone 6276 1380.

UAE

BioCare supplements (see above) are available in Dubai from Organic Foods & Café, PO Box 117629, Dubai, United Arab Emirates, contact +971 44340577.

Index